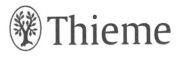

Optimizing Suboptimal Results Following Cataract Surgery

Refractive and Non-Refractive Management

Priya Narang, MS
Director
Narang Eye Care and Laser Centre
Ahmedabad, Gujarat, India

William B. Trattler, MD
Director of Cornea
The Center for Excellence in Eye Care
Volunteer Faculty
Florida International University College of Medicine
Miami, Florida

142 illustrations

Thieme
New York • Stuttgart • Delhi • Rio de Janeiro

Executive Editor: William Lamsback
Managing Editor: Elizabeth Palumbo
Director, Editorial Services: Mary Jo Casey
Production Editor: Naamah Schwartz
International Production Director: Andreas Schabert
Editorial Director: Sue Hodgson
International Marketing Director: Fiona Henderson
International Sales Director: Louisa Turrell
Director of Institutional Sales: Adam Bernacki
Senior Vice President and Chief Operating Officer:
  Sarah Vanderbilt
President: Brian D. Scanlan

Library of Congress Cataloging-in-Publication Data
Names: Narang, Priya, editor. | Trattler, Bill, editor.
Title: Optimizing suboptimal results following cataract
  surgery : refractive and non-refrative management /
  [edited by] Priya Narang, William Trattler.
Description: New York : Thieme, [2019] | Includes
bibliographical references.
Identifiers: LCCN 2018025288| ISBN 9781626238954
(hardcover) | ISBN 9781626238961 (eISBN)
Subjects: | MESH: Cataract Extraction--adverse effects |
  Refractive Surgical
Procedures--adverse effects | Treatment Outcome
Classification: LCC RE451 | NLM WW 260 | DDC 617.7/
  42059--dc23 LC record available at
https://lccn.loc.gov/2018025288

© 2019 Thieme Medical Publishers, Inc.

Thieme Publishers New York
333 Seventh Avenue, New York, NY 10001 USA
+1 800 782 3488, customerservice@thieme.com

Thieme Publishers Stuttgart
Rüdigerstrasse 14, 70469 Stuttgart, Germany
+49 [0]711 8931 421, customerservice@thieme.de

Thieme Publishers Delhi
A-12, Second Floor, Sector-2, Noida-201301
Uttar Pradesh, India
+91 120 45 566 00, customerservice@thieme.in

Thieme Publishers Rio de Janeiro, Thieme Publicações Ltda.
Edifício Rodolpho de Paoli, 25º andar
Av. Nilo Peçanha, 50 – Sala 2508
Rio de Janeiro 20020-906 Brasil
+55 21 3172-2297 / +55 21 3172-1896
www.thiemerevinter.com.br

Cover design: Thieme Publishing Group
Typesetting by Thomson Digital, India

Printed in The United States of America by
King Printing Company, Inc.   5 4 3 2 1

ISBN 978-1-62623-895-4

Also available as an e-book:
eISBN 978-1-62623-896-1

Important note: Medicine is an ever-changing science undergoing continual development. Research and clinical experience are continually expanding our knowledge, in particular our knowledge of proper treatment and drug therapy. Insofar as this book mentions any dosage or application, readers may rest assured that the authors, editors, and publishers have made every effort to ensure that such references are in accordance with **the state of knowledge at the time of production of the book.**

Nevertheless, this does not involve, imply, or express any guarantee or responsibility on the part of the publishers in respect to any dosage instructions and forms of applications stated in the book. **Every user is requested to examine carefully** the manufacturers' leaflets accompanying each drug and to check, if necessary in consultation with a physician or specialist, whether the dosage schedules mentioned therein or the contraindications stated by the manufacturers differ from the statements made in the present book. Such examination is particularly important with drugs that are either rarely used or have been newly released on the market. Every dosage schedule or every form of application used is entirely at the user's own risk and responsibility. The authors and publishers request every user to report to the publishers any discrepancies or inaccuracies noticed. If errors in this work are found after publication, errata will be posted at www.thieme.com on the product description page.

Some of the product names, patents, and registered designs referred to in this book are in fact registered trademarks or proprietary names even though specific reference to this fact is not always made in the text. Therefore, the appearance of a name without designation as proprietary is not to be construed as a representation by the publisher that it is in the public domain.

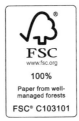

FSC
www.fsc.org
100%
Paper from well-managed forests
FSC® C103101

I would like to dedicate the book to my beautiful, talented daughter **Rhea** who too aspires to be an ophthalmologist one day. I am also thankful to my family for being my strength and for their continued support and love throughout the writing of the book and also within my life as they have helped me in more ways than anyone else.

Priya Narang

I dedicate this book to my parents, Marcia and Henry, who both make such a difference to their friends and family. Their positive energy and zest for making a difference have been inspirational. I am very grateful, and I hope that I can carry on their kindness, compassion and positive outlook on life.

William B. Trattler

Contents

Part I Introduction

Part II Refractive Enhancement Procedures

Video Contents

Foreword

A generation ago, the first step in refractive cataract surgery began when we routinely began to implant intraocular lenses (IOLs) to provide visual rehabilitation for the management of aphakia in the cataract surgery patient. Today, the opportunities for these same cataract surgical patients have expanded dramatically with the next generation of refractive cataract surgery. Multifocal, extended depth of field, toric, accommodating, and aspheric IOLs have improved visual quality and empowered us with additional opportunities to meet our patients' needs. However, the IOL is only a portion of the cataract surgical procedure. We continue to advance our profession by improving the safety and accuracy of cataract surgery as well. Accuracy has been improved with the addition of better keratometry, biometry, posterior cornea evaluation, and IOL formulas. Our most challenging and often our most demanding patients are those who have undergone previous corneal refractive surgery and have an increased expectation of excellent uncorrected visual acuity. Intraocular aberrometry has been a major advance for these difficult IOL calculations as well as for improving accuracy of toric IOL implantation. When there is residual refractive error following cataract surgery, astigmatic keratotomy, LASIK (laser in situ keratomileusis), PRK (photorefractive keratectomy), IOL exchange, piggyback IOLs, and in the near future light-adjustable IOLs are all viable options to resolve the refractive error. Safety has also increased as we have become more proficient in managing the most difficult surgical cases with the aid of better techniques and technology. However, serious complications such as endophthalmitis and retinal detachment continue to occur, but with precautions these complications can be reduced. Dry eye, while rarely vision threatening, is the single most common complication associated with cataract surgery, and recent advances in the diagnosis and treatment of this disorder have dramatically improved patient satisfaction following cataract surgery.

As patient expectations have increased, there is more of a need today than ever before to improve our surgical outcomes and to address the patient whose expectations have not been met. The true measure of a successful cataract surgeon is not how he or she treats the happy surgical patient but how they prevent complications, increase the quality of surgical outcomes, and most importantly resolve the issues that result in an unhappy cataract surgery patient. This is the core message of *Optimizing Suboptimal Results Following Cataract Surgery*. There are several important steps that, when executed correctly, dramatically increase postoperative success with refractive IOL cataract surgery. In general, cataract surgery, and more specifically premium IOL cataract surgery, requires careful patient selection and counseling, along with precise surgical technique. The preoperative evaluation is extraordinarily important to determine which lens is best for a specific patient. High hyperopia, myopia, corneal disease, concomitant glaucoma, and previous vitreoretinal disease all create unique challenges for the cataract surgeon. Recent design advances in IOLs have resulted in excellent visual outcomes after cataract surgery. As a result, many patients now have higher expectations for vision following surgery, including complete spectacle independence.

Priya Narang and William Trattler are two of the unique thinkers of our time in the field of ophthalmic anterior segment surgery. There is an enormous unmet need for a book that addresses the prevention and management of the suboptimal surgical result in the cataract patient. This unmet need has been answered with this book, *Optimizing Suboptimal Results Following Cataract Surgery*. The challenges cataract surgeons deal with every day are presented by Drs. Narang and Trattler and their superlative faculty to give every ophthalmologist the opportunity to learn from the best and to enhance their surgical results. This book is founded on the basic principle that the patient always comes first and we should do everything to maximize their visual outcome. No case is too complex for the carefully selected international faculty of skilled ophthalmic surgeons who are authors in this book.

Optimizing Suboptimal Results Following Cataract Surgery is a comprehensive analysis of the advances in the field of cataract surgery that improve patient outcomes. It summarizes all of the best, most useful, and practical pearls that have been recently developed and gives the reader a glimpse of the future of refractive cataract surgery. Drs. Narang and Trattler are to be congratulated for bringing together an internationally recognized group of authors and a comprehensive series of videos to demonstrate their most useful techniques. There is no surgical procedure that improves quality of life with greater efficacy than modern cataract surgery. This book delivers to its readers the experience of leading ophthalmic surgeons on how to realize the promise of refractive cataract surgery and will be widely read and appreciated by anterior segment surgeons who wish to add to their surgical armamentarium and will be an important contribution to ophthalmology.

Eric Donnenfeld, MD
Clinical Professor of Ophthalmology
New York University Medical Center
Trustee, Dartmouth Medical School
Immediate Past President, ASCRS

Preface

The editors are delighted to present their joint venture entitled *Optimizing Suboptimal Results Following Cataract Surgery: Refractive and Non-Refractive Management*. The book has been written and presented with the concept of highlighting the suboptimal outcomes that follow a cataract surgery, which may serve as a major disappointment to the surgeon as well as the patient. The unique feature of the book is that it serves as a concise review and as a comprehensive guide on the concerned topic for all the ophthalmologists, residents, and fellows along with subspecialists. The book focuses on the aspect of untutored and unversed technicality that is an essential and an indispensable knowledge tool for the operating surgeon, and it brings to the forefront the arsenal of discreet medical facts.

The book has 23 chapters with illustrative details authored by renowned ophthalmologists who are specialized in their respective field of handling the clinical challenges. In addition to this, the book is also accompanied by surgical videos that serve as an additional valuable learning tool.

We deeply appreciate the generous efforts of all the authors and contributors in enabling us to pursue the completion of the book.

Priya Narang, MS
William B. Trattler, MD

Contributors

Amar Agarwal, MS, FRCS, FRCOphthal
Chairman
Dr. Agarwal's Group of Eye Hospitals and Eye
  Research Centre
Chennai, India

Jorge L. Alió, MD
Professor and Chairman of Ophthalmology
Miguel Hernandez University
Alicante, Spain

Renato Ambrósio Jr., MD, PhD
Founder
Rio de Janeiro Corneal Tomography and
  Biomechanics Study Group
Professor of Ophthalmology
Federal University of The State of Rio de
  Janeiro (UNIRIO)
Federal University of São Paulo (UNIFESP)
Clinical Director
Insistuto de Olhos Renato Ambrósio
VisareRIO
Refracta Perosnal Laser
Rio de Janeiro, Brazil

Eric Clayton Amesbury, MD
Staff Ophthalmologist
Veterans Administration Medical Center
Assistant Professor of Ophthalmology
Medical College of Virginia
Virginia Commonwealth University
Richmond, Virginia

Fernando A. Arevalo, BS
Student
Clinica Oftalmologica Centro Caracas
Caracas, Venezuela

J. Fernando Arevalo, MD, FACS
Edmund F. and Virginia B. Ball Professor
  of Ophthalmology
Chairman
Department of Ophthalmology
Johns Hopkins Bayview Medical Center
Retina Division, Wilmer Eye Institute
The Johns Hopkins University School of Medicine
Baltimore, Maryland

Jacqueline Beltz, FRANZCO
Staff Specialist Ophthalmologist
Centre for Eye Research Australia
Royal Victorian Eye and Ear Hospital
East Melbourne, Victoria, Australia

Lisa Y. Chen, MD
Clinical Instructor
Department of Ophthalmology
Byers Eye Institute at Stanford
Stanford University School of Medicine
Palo Alto, California

**Arthur B. Cummings, MMed (Ophth),
  FCS(SA), FRCSEd**
Medical Director
Wellington Eye Clinic
Department Head
Beacon Hospital
Dublin, Ireland

**Sheraz Daya, MD, FACP, FACS, FRCS(Ed),
  FRCOphth**
Medical Director
Centre for Sight
East Grinstead, West Sussex, United Kingdom

Uday Devgan, MD, FACS FRCS
Private Practice
Devgan Eye Surgery
Los Angeles, California
Partner
Specialty Surgical Center
Beverly Hills, California
Chief of Ophthalmology
Olive View UCLA Medical Center
Los Angeles, California
Clinical Professor of Ophthalmology
Jules Stein Eye Institute
UCLA School of Medicine
Los Angeles, California

Fernando Antonio Faria-Correia, MD, PhD
Ophthalmologiest
CUF Porto
Oftalconde, Porto, Portugal
Hospital de Braga
Escola de Medicina da Universidade do Minho
Braga, Portugal
Rio de Janeiro Corneal Tomography and Biomechanics
    Study Group
Rio de Janeiro, Brazil

Carlos F. Fernández, MD
Director
Vitreo Retinal Service Clinica Oftalmologica
    Oftalmolaser
Santiago de Surco, Lima, Peru

Nicole R. Fram, MD
Clinical Instructor
David Geffen School of Medicine
UCLA Stein Eye Institute
Advanced Vision Care
Los Angeles, California

Johnny L. Gayton, MD
Chief Medical Officer
Gayton Health Centre
Warner Robins, Georgia

Andrzej Grzybowski, MD, PhD, MBA
Professor of Ophthalmology
Department Head of Ophthalmology
Poznan, Poland
Chair of Ophthalmology
University of Warmia and Mazury
Olsztyn, Poland

Kathryn M. Hatch, MD
Director
Refractive Surgery Service
Massachusetts Eye & Ear
Site Director
Massachusetts Eye & Ear Waltham
Assistant Professor of Ophthalmology
Harvard Medical School
Boston, Massachusetts

Tsontcho Ianchulev, MD, MPH
Professor of Ophthalmology
New York Eye and Ear Infirmary
Icahn School of Medicine New York
New York, New York

Jonathan K. Kam, MBBS (Hons), BMedSc (Hons)
Advanced Cataract Fellow
Surgical Ophthalmology Service
Royal Victorian Eye and Ear Hospital
East Melbourne, Victoria, Australia

Isaac Lipshitz, MD
CEO, Medical Director
OptoLight Vision
Herzlia, Israel

Jennifer Loh, MD
Founder
Loh Ophthalmology
Board Member
Eye Physicians of Florida
Volunteer Faculty
Larkin Hospital Ophthalmology Residency Program
Miami, Florida

Susan MacDonald, MD
Associate Professor of Ophthalmology
Tufts School of Medicine
Lahey Clinic Medical Centre
Concord, Massachusetts

Edward E. Manche, MD
Director of Cornea and Refractive Surgery
Byers Eye Institute
Professor of Ophthalmology
Stanford University School of Medicine
Palo Alto, California

Samuel Masket, MD
Clinical Professor
David Geffen School of Medicine
UCLA Stein Eye Institute
Founding Partner
Advanced Vision Care
Los Angeles, California

José Carlos Ferreira Mendes, MD
Ophthalmologist
Department of Ophthalmology
Hospital de Braga
PT School of Medicine
Universidade do Minho
Braga, Portugal

Kevin M. Miller, MD
Kolokotrones Chair in Ophthalmology
Chief
Cataract and Refractive Surgery Division
Director
Anterior Segment Diagnostic Laboratory
David Geffen School of Medicine and UCLA
Los Angeles, California

Priya Narang, MS
Director
Narang Eye Care and Laser Center
Ahmedabad, Gujarat, India

Samir Narang, MS, DO
Director
Narang Eye Hospital
Ahmedabad, Gujarat, India

Thomas A. Oetting, MD
Rudy and Margaret Perez Professor of Ophthalmology
Director
Ophthalmology Residency Program
University of Iowa
Iowa City, Iowa

Laura M. Periman, MD
Ophthalmologist
Redmond Eye Clinic
Redmond, Washington

Mario J. Rojas, MD
Resident
Eastern Virginia Medical School
Norfolk, Virginia

Riley N. Sanders, MD
Resident
University for Arkansas for Medical Sciences
The Jones Eye Institute
Outpatient Circle
Little Rock, Arkansas

Val Nordin Sanders, CRA, COT
Technical Consultant
Gayton Health Centre
Warner Robins, Georgia

Aazim A. Siddiqui, MD
Resident Physician
Department of Ophthalmology and Visual Sciences
Montefiore Medical Center
Albert Einstein College of Medicine
New York, New York

William B. Trattler, MD
Director of Cornea
The Center for Excellence in Eye Care
Volunteer Faculty
Florida International University College of Medicine
Miami, Florida

Magdalena Turczynowska, MD
Ophthalmologist
Stefan Zeromski Specialist
Municipal Hospital in Krakow
Krakow, Poland

Veronica Vargas Fragoso, MD
Ophthalmologist
Refractive Surgery Fellow
Department of Investigation
Development and Innovation
Vissum Alicante, Spain

Gary Wörtz, MD
Ophthalmologist
Commonwealth Eye Surgery
Associate Professor of Ophthalmology
University of Kentucky, College of Medicine
Chief Medical Officer
Omega Ophthalmics
Lexington, Kentucky

Elizabeth Yeu, MD
Assistant Professor of Ophthalmology
Eastern Virginia Medical School
Norfolk, Virginia

Part I

Introduction

1 Overview of the Causes of Suboptimal Outcomes Following Cataract Surgery: Role of Preoperative Screening and Adequate Counseling

Samir Narang and Priya Narang

Abstract

The causes of suboptimal outcomes following a cataract surgery can range from tear film abnormality to posterior segment disorder. Adequate preoperative screening and proper counseling help achieve an optimal result that eventually builds up the doctor–patient relationship to a satisfied and happy patient.

Keywords: preoperative screening, suboptimal outcomes, cataract screening, counseling, specular microscopy, informed consent

1.1 Overview of the Causes of Suboptimal Outcomes

There can be varied causes for suboptimal outcomes after cataract surgery that on a broad spectrum can range from the instability of tear film to corneal involvement and disorders, intraoperative inflammation, raised intraocular pressure (IOP) to vitreoretinal, and optic nerve involvement to a more serious condition such as endophthalmitis. On a lighter note, it can be an error of wrong intraocular lens (IOL) power calculation and insertion of a wrong IOL although the repercussions of this are quite serious as it leads to residual refractive error, and especially in the era of premium IOL surgeries, patients' expectations are quite high and the surgeon has a constant challenge to meet these expectations. However, with the involvement of each layer or tissue of an eye in a detailed and multiple ways, the cause for suboptimal outcomes can be multiple. All the potential causes and preexisting ocular comorbidities should be diagnosed and evaluated, and the prospective outcomes should be discussed with the patient.

1.2 Preoperative Screening

Preoperative screening and examination although a routine is an essential prerequisite before surgical procedures that helps stratify risk, direct anesthetic choices, and guide the postoperative management.

The preoperative screening is guided by the patient's clinical history, comorbidities, and physical examination findings. This decision is multifactorial and involves consideration of visual status: individual patient's vision requirements, patient motivation, ability of the eye to withstand surgical stresses, and the motivation or desire of the patient to proceed with a surgical option.

Although there is one treatment option for cataract, the complexity is multifold in a way from choosing the right IOL to the right IOL calculation formula, from preexisting retinal disorders to compromised endothelium, and from complexity of diagnostic tests to the risk of significant complications or comorbidities that may lead to suboptimal cataract surgery outcomes.

1.3 History Evaluation

1.3.1 Medical/Metabolic Illness

Proper medical history evaluation of the patient is essential, and leading questions from the surgeon asking for any systemic illness such as hypertension, diabetes (▶ Fig. 1.1), thyroid disorder, cardiac, or any other disorder for which the patient needs

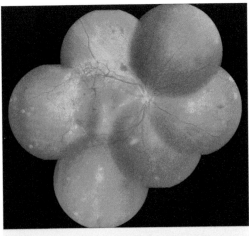

Fig. 1.1 Fundus image of diabetic retinopathy.

to take any medicine should be evaluated. In males above 50 years of age, leading question of any drug consumed for prostate enlargement should be asked for as it can lead to intraoperative floppy iris syndrome. Anticoagulants and blood-thinning agents should be stopped at least 3 to 4 days before the surgery is planned and can be resumed once the surgery is over.

Metabolic or genetic disorder history also carries a lot of weightage as it helps the surgeon to specifically look for the signs of the disorder. For example, for all cases of Marfan's or Weil–Marchesani syndrome, the zonular integrity should be carefully assessed even though there is no major lenticular dislocation at the time of preoperative examination. This helps evade any unpleasant intraoperative surprise and apprises the surgeon of the correct ocular status.

History of any previous refractive or ocular surgery should also be evaluated. In case of history of refractive surgery, proper preoperative evaluation is again needed as to the calculation of the IOL power by applying appropriate IOL power calculation formulas after taking all the aspects into consideration. In cases with higher or asymmetric refractive errors in both the eyes, amblyopia should be ruled out and possible causes and outcomes should be evaluated.

Detailed history about the visual status of the patient few years ago can go miles in explaining the preoperative status of the eye.

History of previous retinal surgery or an intravitreal injection should draw a cataract surgeon's attention to the aspect of performing a cataract surgery in previtrectomized eyes and the possibility of an increase incidence of intraoperative posterior capsular rupture.[1,2,3,4,5,6,7] Previous intravitreal injections have the probability of damaging the posterior capsule and a preoperative B-scan or, if possible, an optical coherence tomography (OCT) examination to assess the integrity of the posterior capsule should be performed.

1.4 Vision

Recording visual acuity helps evaluate the functional visual capacity of the patient who is to undergo a surgery. The fall in vision should be correlated to the degree of cataract in the eye, and in case the functional vision loss exceeds the degree of cataract, other causes must be evaluated for the relevant fall of visual capacity.

1.5 Ocular Motility and Alignment Analysis

Squint analysis should always be performed and microtropia should always be assessed as it directs an underlying cause of amblyopia that may be present in a cataractous eye. Assessment of ocular motility should always be done to rule out any paralytic component. In addition to this, cover–uncover test, assessment of head posture, detection of cyclotorsion, or any associated nystagmus should also be performed.

1.6 Specular Microscopy and Pachymetry

Specular microscope (► Fig. 1.2a) helps detect corneal endotheliopathy (► Fig. 1.2b; ► Fig. 1.3) and forms an essential component of preoperative screening before a cataract surgery. A normal cataract surgery leads to 4 to 10% of the endothelial cell density (ECD) loss following surgery. This loss can be more in cases with preexisting endotheliopathies with less ECD count. Additionally, constant use of contact lens wear along with previous intraocular surgery also has a detrimental effect on the corneal endothelium. Assessment of all these corneal conditions helps determine a treatment plan for cases with diseased endothelium. Low ECD counts (► Fig. 1.3) with distorted ECD morphology invoke the application of endothelium-saving strategies that prevent further cell loss.

Patients with diseases such as glaucoma, iridocyclitis, or diabetes, or with history of previous ocular surgery are at increased risk of ECD loss and its adverse effects on cornea postsurgery (► Fig. 1.4). In accordance with specular microscopy, pachymetry should also be performed to assess the corneal thickness in eyes with compromised corneas.

1.7 Intraocular Lens Power Calculation and Intraocular Lens Choices

Essential preoperative testing includes keratometry readings, ultrasound axial length of the eye (A-scan), corneal topographic scanning, and a calculation of implant power requirements using a modern implant formula. Optional testing also might include potential visual acuity testing and ophthalmic photography.

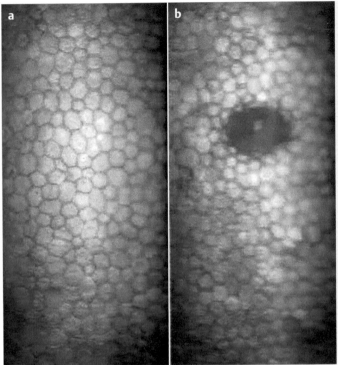

Fig. 1.2 Specular microscopy images. **(a)** Specular microscope denoting the normal endothelial cell count, shape, and morphology. **(b)** Scattered guttata seen, suggesting possibility of development of early Fuch's syndrome. (These images are provided courtesy of Dr. Ashish Nagpal, Retina Foundation, Ahmedabad, India.)

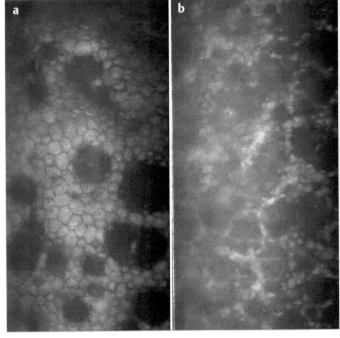

Fig. 1.3 Fuchs' dystrophy. **(a)** Moderate Fuch's dystrophy. **(b)** Advanced Fuch's dystrophy with endotheliopathy. (These images are provided courtesy of Dr. Ashish Nagpal, Retina Foundation, Ahmedabad, India.)

Patients who have undergone a silicon oil implantation may give erroneous readings while performing IOL power calculation. All measures should be taken to counteract this error by employing the conversion factor during IOL power calculation. The conversion factor of 0.71 corrects for an apparent increase in axial length induced by silicon oil of viscosity 1,300 cSt.[8]

While implanting IOLs in such cases, silicon IOL should be deferred and a lens with 360-degree square edge with large optic diameter of 6 to 6.5 mm should be preferred as it gives greater viewing area for fundus examination.

1.8 Pupillary Reflexes and Posterior Segment Examination

Pupillary reflexes should be elicited in all the cases as it gives a correct idea of the status of the optic nerve and its pathway. This is especially important in hard and brunescent cataracts where it is difficult to evaluate the fundus due to increased density of the nucleus. A relative pupillary afferent defect in such circumstances indicates pathology in the posterior segment and a B-scan should be impertinently performed to rule out the anomaly.

The goal of preoperative fundus examination is to recognize any finding of clinical significance with regard to correct choice of the surgical procedure. Any finding of clinical significance is recorded on a fundus chart in all cases (▶ Fig. 1.5, ▶ Fig. 1.6, ▶ Fig. 1.7). The importance of performing a B-scan and an OCT wherever possible cannot be underestimated as it often leads to detection of subtle signs of retinal and macular disorders that maybe preexisting due to any other associated pathology or may exist as a separate entity (▶ Fig. 1.8; ▶ Fig. 1.9). Nevertheless, fundus photography (▶ Fig. 1.10) and OCT examination help

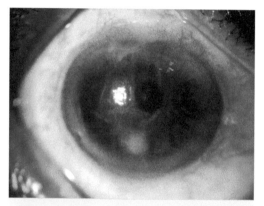

Fig. 1.4 Postoperative bullous keratopathy in a compromised cornea with low endothelial cell count.

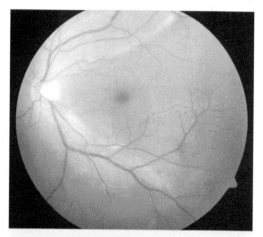

Fig. 1.6 Retinal detachment.

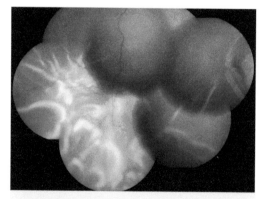

Fig. 1.5 Retinal detachment.

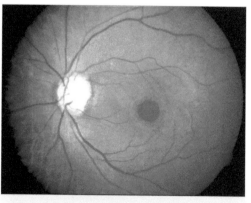

Fig. 1.7 Fundus examination demonstrating full-thickness macular hole.

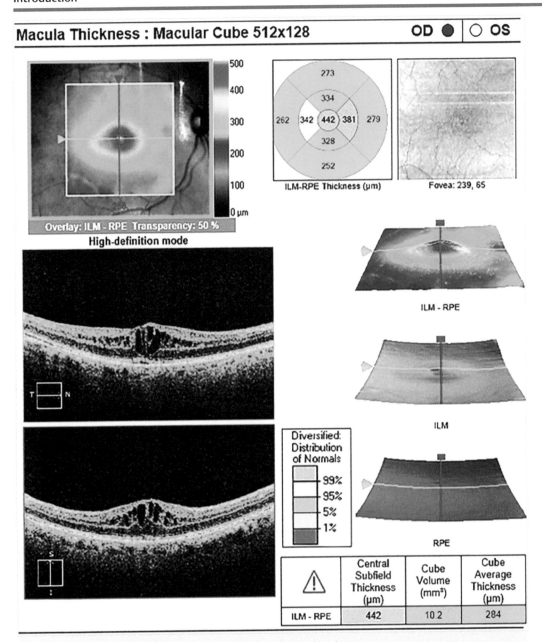

Fig. 1.8 Optical coherence tomography demonstrating cystoid macular edema.

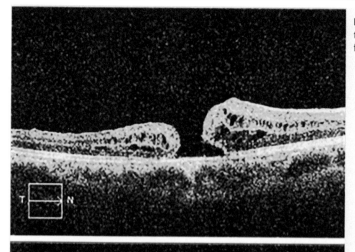

Fig. 1.9 Optical coherence tomography demonstrating full-thickness macular hole.

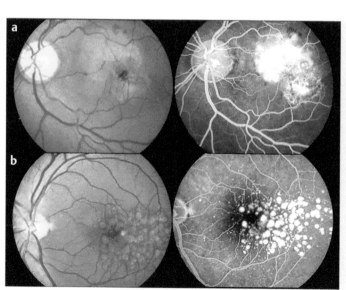

Fig. 1.10 Age-related macular degeneration (ARMD). **(a)** Fundus photograph and fluorescein angiography of wet ARMD. **(b)** Fundus photograph and fluorescein angiography of dry ARMD.

document the preexisting pathology and also help explain to the patient about the potential limitations that will ensue in the postoperative recovery period.

1.9 Intraocular Pressure

Proper preoperative IOP charting gives a clear insight into the possibility of the involvement of visual fields. In case of suspicion, gonioscopy should be performed to assess the angle structures, and visual field perimetry along with optic disc analysis should be done.

1.10 Laboratory Investigations

Preoperative blood sugar assessment forms a very crucial test for a patient undergoing cataract surgery. Apart from this, the importance of getting other lab examinations such as a routine blood count, coagulation studies, or chest radiography depends on the associated features that the patient presents with and the comorbidities. It also depends a lot on the type of anesthesia that the patient is being administered. A complete set of detailed preoperative workup is essential for patients undergoing a general anesthesia for surgery, whereas a less detailed workup will be necessary for a patient undergoing a peribulbar block. Moreover, the set of preoperative lab examinations also depends a lot on the health care system of the country that the surgeon practices from.

1.11 Informed Consent and Role of Counseling

Counseling a patient helps set a realistic approach toward the surgical outcomes and especially in eyes or cases where suboptimal outcome is anticipated. Patients having low ECD count should be made to understand their physiological alteration that is preexisting and the possible postoperative outcomes. They should also be informed about the complications that can arise due to low ECD in spite of all intraoperative precautions.

Each patient needs a customized approach as the requirements and expectations of each patient vary. The type of IOL that is best suited to the patient's need should be advised with the possible limitations and advantages.

Preoperative workup with proper counseling heralds a better doctor–patient relationship as both aim at the practical and achievable targets with realistic expectations and possible constraints.

1.12 Key Pearls

- Adequate preoperative screening is an essential part of examination for patients scheduled for cataract surgery.
- Personal as well as family history evaluation adds significant information and guides the surgeon to the possibility of various clinical conditions that may be associated with cataract and that may influence the surgery.
- In cases of hard cataract, where fundus and OCT evaluation of the posterior segment is difficult, pupillary reflexes should be elicited that give a brief overview of the optic nerve conduction and of the retinal status.
- Setting up a realistic goal and helping the patient to understand the clinical scenario with all the pros and cons of the surgery is extremely important to have a happy patient in the postoperative period.

References

[1] Blankenship GW, Machemer R. Long-term diabetic vitrectomy results. Report of 10 year follow-up. Ophthalmology. 1985; 92(4):503–506

[2] Biró Z, Kovács B. Results of cataract surgery in previously vitrectomized eyes. J Cataract Refract Surg. 2002; 28(6): 1003–1006

[3] Chang MA, Parides MK, Chang S, Braunstein RE. Outcome of phacoemulsification after pars plana vitrectomy. Ophthalmology. 2002; 109(5):948–954

[4] Díaz Lacalle V, Orbegozo Gárate FJ, Martinez Alday N, López Garrido JA, Aramberri Agesta J. Phacoemulsification cataract surgery in vitrectomized eyes. J Cataract Refract Surg. 1998; 24(6):806–809

[5] Pinter SM, Sugar A. Phacoemulsification in eyes with past pars plana vitrectomy: case-control study. J Cataract Refract Surg. 1999; 25(4):556–561

[6] Grusha YO, Masket S, Miller KM. Phacoemulsification and lens implantation after pars plana vitrectomy. Ophthalmology. 1998; 105(2):287–294

[7] Ahfat FG, Yuen CHW, Groenewald CP. Phacoemulsification and intraocular lens implantation following pars plana vitrectomy: a prospective study. Eye (Lond). 2003; 17(1): 16–20

[8] Murray DC, Durrani OM, Good P, Benson MT, Kirkby GR. Biometry of the silicone oil-filled eye: II. Eye (Lond). 2002; 16 (6):727–730

2 Tear Film and Corneal Disorders

Laura M. Periman and Priya Narang

Abstract

This chapter touches upon a select few of the myriad contributors to postoperative refraction inaccuracies including the visual and keratometric impacts of a compromised tear film as well as the visual contributions and consequences of corneal disorders in the cataract surgery setting.

Keywords: cataract refractive outcomes, IOL selection, CDED, OSD, osmolarity, keratometry, keratometric errors, IOL calculation errors, wound healing, corneal nerves, growth factors, wavefront, aberrometry, scatter

2.1 Introduction

Despite advanced equipment, sophisticated formulae, and significant surgeon effort in choosing the ideal intraocular lens (IOL) power, postcataract surgical refractive outcomes are not as precise as we desire and expect. Crowdsourced online super formulae have improved predictability such that approximately 90% of cases result in refractive outcomes ±0.5 diopters of target refraction.

Myriad dynamic and static factors contribute to suboptimal cataract surgery results. Two broad categories of topics will be used to review common and clinically significant factors that contribute to suboptimal post cataract outcomes: tear film disorders and corneal disorders.

2.2 Tear Film Disorders

The most common tear film disorder is chronic dry eye disease (CDED; ▶ Fig. 2.1). The Tear Film & Ocular Surface (TFOS)/Dry Eye Workshop II (DEWS II) report[1] provides a complete scientific literature review and consensus-based organization of the current state of knowledge on dry eye. Trattler et al[2] found in a multicenter prospective study that approximately 80% of patients presenting for cataract surgery had evidence of CDED. Additionally, 50% had central corneal staining, which would be associated with backward light scatter as a contributor to subjective blur, discussed later.[2,3] CDED impacts preoperative keratometry,[4] IOL calculations,

and postsurgical visual performance as well as patient satisfaction and quality of life.[1]

2.2.1 Optical Aberrations: Higher Order Aberrations and Light Scatter as Mechanisms of Visual Disturbance in CDED

Standard high-contrast visual acuity testing is inadequate for exploring and understanding the quality of visual performance. Recent technological advances in devices such as wavefront analysis and point spread function analysis capture visual quality and provide insight into the dissatisfied 20/20 postoperative cataract patient. As reviewed by Koh,[3] analysis of optical performance can help bridge the gaps in the sign/symptom disconnect in CDED.

Light scatter can occur as forward or as backward light scatter. With respect to CDED, both phenomena occur and can be used to help explain suboptimal subjective visual complaints. Koh reported the amount of anterior or forward light scatter is statistically significantly higher for CDED with unstable tear film (rapid tear breakup time, or TBUT) and also for CDED with superficial punctate keratopathy (SPK) compared to normal individuals. Forward light scatter contributes to subjective glare. However, posterior light scatter is associated with subjective blur and is statistically significantly worse only in SPK and not with rapid TBUT. Higher order aberrations in wavefront

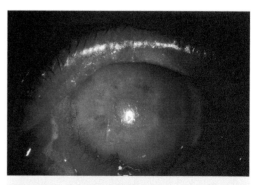

Fig. 2.1 Case of chronic dry eye disease. (This image is provided courtesy of Sonal Tuli.)

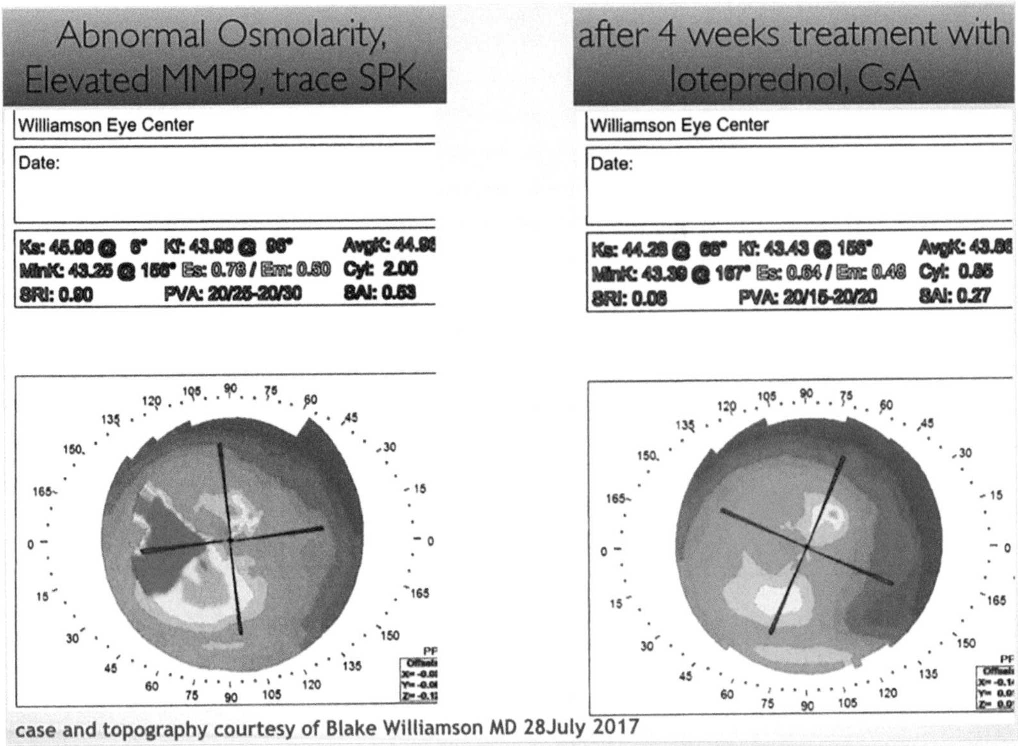

> **Abnormal Osmolarity, Elevated MMP9, trace SPK**
>
> Williamson Eye Center
>
> Date:
>
> Ka: 45.96 @ 6° Kf: 43.96 @ 96° AvgK: 44.96
> MinK: 43.25 @ 156° Es: 0.78 / Em: 0.50 Cyl: 2.00
> SRI: 0.80 PVA: 20/25-20/30 SAI: 0.63

> **after 4 weeks treatment with loteprednol, CsA**
>
> Williamson Eye Center
>
> Date:
>
> Ka: 44.28 @ 66° Kf: 43.43 @ 156° AvgK: 43.86
> MinK: 43.39 @ 167° Es: 0.64 / Em: 0.48 Cyl: 0.85
> SRI: 0.08 PVA: 20/15-20/20 SAI: 0.27

case and topography courtesy of Blake Williamson MD 28July 2017

Fig. 2.2 Topographic and keratometric maps demonstrating the impact of hyperosmolarity associated with inflammation and chronic dry eye disease. Note the changes in topography, keratometry values as well as axis of astigmatism. Patient was interested in a premium intraocular lens (IOL). If a toric IOL had been calculated based off the first readings, cylinder overcorrection and incorrect axis placement would have resulted as well as a 1.0-diopter postcataract refractive error. (Case and image provided courtesy of Blake Williamson, July 28, 2017.)

analysis contribute to blur and fluctuations. Eye fatigue encompasses glare, blur, and fluctuations.

2.2.2 Keratometric Aberrations

A healthy ocular surface is under homeostatic control of the lacrimal functional unit. A healthy system is designed to withstand environmental, traumatic, and microbial insults by mounting a stress response and an amplification response while also modulating a damage and repair/remodeling phase before finally returning to homeostatic control.[1] With CDED, homeostasis-maintaining mechanisms and signals are compromised, resulting in a chronically activated stress response (nuclear factor-κB, mitogen-activated protein kinase, interleukin-1 [IL-1], tumor necrosis factor [TNF]) and chronically elevated damage phase (IL-17, g-IFN-γ, TNF-α), which leads to damage to the goblet cells, epithelium, and sub-basal corneal nerve plexus. IL-1 and TNF induce nerve growth factor (NGF) from the human limbal basal epithelium. When NGF is chronically upregulated in response to CDED, corneal nerve dysmorphology and epithelial cell apoptosis occur via high-affinity and low-affinity NGF receptors, respectively. Recent confocal microscopy evidence indicates that epithelial cell density, keratocyte activation, and corneal nerve dysmorphology improve after 6 months of treatment with topical cyclosporine A.[5] This has implications for an appropriate postoperative wound and nerve healing response.

2.2.3 Visual Performance and Patient Satisfaction

Visual performance is subjective; however, optical analysis can provide objective insight as discussed earlier. Data gathered from the Progression of Ocular Findings (PROOF) study[6] (designed to study the natural history of progression of CDED) indicate a significant component of subjective visual fluctuations

(57.6%) in level 2 CDED patients compared to controls (10.5%) despite 20/20 vision (PROOF). CDED is increasingly considered a vision disease. The literature also indicates a significant impact of CDED on keratometric repeatability,[4] which can induce IOL calculation errors and thereby affect postoperative refractive outcomes (▶ Fig. 2.2). Additionally, patient satisfaction, visual performance, productivity and quality of life are impacted by CDED.[1] Arguably, all of these factors are potentially implicated in suboptimal results following cataract surgery.

2.3 Corneal Disorders

Irrespective of the density of the corneal lesion, the visual output is always compromised in patients with corneal disorders and the status is worse when the visual axis is affected. The corneal lesion can be an old healed scar due to either trauma or keratitis or it may range from corneal degeneration (▶ Fig. 2.3) to corneal dystrophy (▶ Fig. 2.4, ▶ Fig. 2.5) or may even have medication toxicity (▶ Fig. 2.6). The etiology of the type of corneal lesion should be identified as it helps guide the patient about the possible outcomes following cataract surgery.

Postsurgery, the lesion of viral keratitis may become activated and the patient might need an additional therapy of viral keratitis with antiviral drugs. Patients with leucomatous corneal opacity or with progressive degeneration or dystrophy might need a corneal transplant to optimize their visual outcome.

Patients with low endothelial cell density (ECD) count or with Fuch's dystrophy should have the endothelium well coated with suitable ophthalmic viscosurgical device that prevents endothelial cell loss to prevent hastening the need for a corneal transplant. In addition to this, the choice of cataract procedure should also be chosen wisely so as to minimally disturb the ECD. In cases with low ECD counts and dense cataracts, an extra capsular cataract extraction (ECCE) procedure or a manual

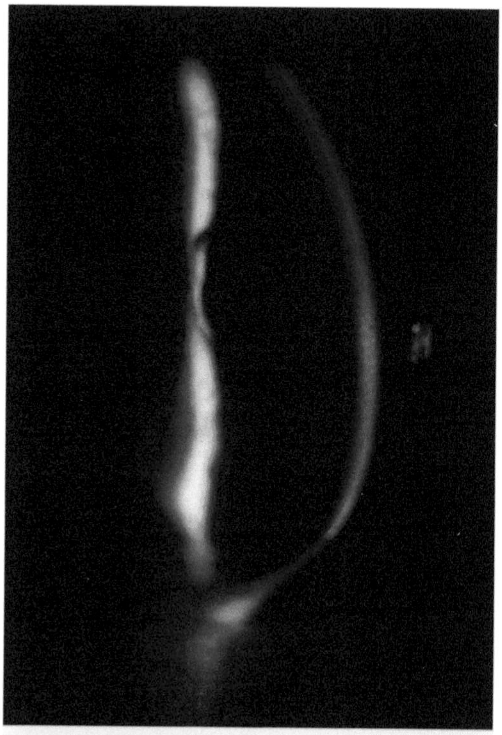

Fig. 2.3 Pellucid marginal degeneration. (This image is provided courtesy of Sonal Tuli.)

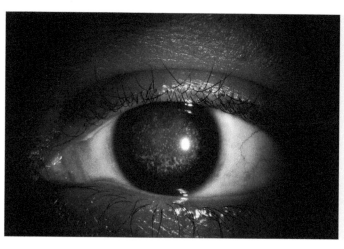

Fig. 2.4 Granular corneal dystrophy. (This image is provided courtesy of Sonal Tuli.)

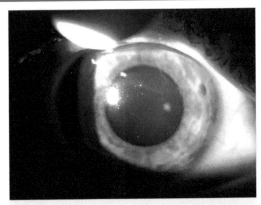

Fig. 2.6 Medication toxicity. (This image is provided courtesy of Sonal Tuli.)

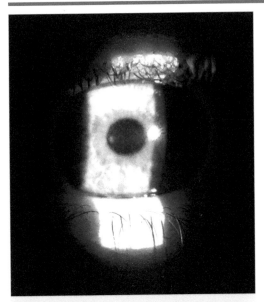

Fig. 2.5 Bowman's dystrophy. (This image is provided courtesy of Sonal Tuli.)

small-incision cataract surgery (SICS) should be performed, which prevents ECD loss. The use of high-viscosity viscoelastic, such as Healon GV (sodium hyaluronate), and minimal anterior chamber manipulations may help preserve the endothelium. It may be advisable to perform ECCE, rather than phacoemulsification or manual SICS. In cases with central corneal opacity that obscures the pupil, performing an optical sector iridectomy can be helpful.

In addition to adopting special methods to prevent ECD loss, the patients with corneal disorders also pose a problem for calculation of the keratometry value. In cases of unilateral involvement, the keratometric and axial length measurement of the other eye can serve the purpose, whereas in cases with bilateral corneal involvement, the standard keratometry values of a normal cornea can be taken into consideration.

2.4 Enhancement of the Intraoperative View

With limited intraoperative visualization of the iris, capsule, and lens, performing a successful cataract surgery is in itself a daunting task. Various methods have been suggested to enhance the intraoperative visualization during a cataract surgery that range from the use of oblique illumination to the application of trypan blue dye to stain the anterior capsule to enhance the intraoperative view and contrast.

A standard coaxial lighting mounted on the operating microscopes obscures the surgeon's view due to backscatter and reflection of light from the corneal surface. Habeeb et al[7] described the use of oblique light source in combination with 0.1% trypan blue to improve visualization of the anterior chamber and anterior lens capsule on a patient with severe corneal scarring, whereas Farjo et al[8] described the use of a noninvasive fiberoptic light source to provide oblique illumination without capsular staining and Nishimura et al[9] used a similar technique with indocyanine green to stain the capsulorrhexis, and they then inserted the light source into the eye through a corneal paracentesis to complete phacoemulsification.

Endoilluminator-assisted transcorneal illumination often helps delineate the intraocular details clearly (▶ Fig. 2.7, ▶ Fig. 2.8, ▶ Fig. 2.9, ▶ Fig. 2.10). Adopting these special measures in eyes with pre-existing corneal opacities and low ECD counts helps increase the potential postoperative output in these compromised eyes.

2.5 Conclusion

Visual performance may be compromised by a range of conditions from the pre-corneal tear film to corneal irregularities or conditions involving any of the five corneal layers (▶ Table 2.1).

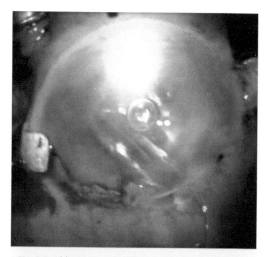

Fig. 2.7 Oblique transcorneal illumination with an endoilluminator enhances the intraoperative view during intraocular lens insertion.

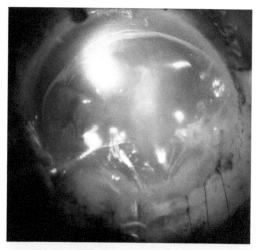

Fig. 2.9 Oblique illumination enhancing the view to perform descemetorhexis in scarred cornea.

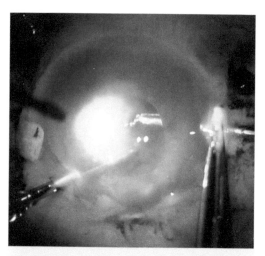

Fig. 2.8 Better haptic visualization with transcorneal illumination during glue-assisted intrascleral fixation procedure.

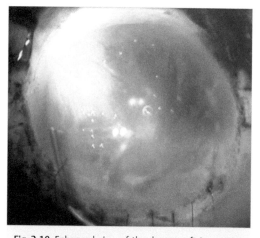

Fig. 2.10 Enhanced view of the donor graft in anterior chamber during endothelial keratoplasty procedure.

Visual acuity and visual performance are intimately related and implicated in cataract surgery outcomes. While emphasis on quantitative visual acuity remains, new methods for understanding qualitative visual performance have the potential to provide greater insight into suboptimal cataract outcomes.

2.6 Key Pearls

- **Pursue:** hunt for clues suggesting the presence of ocular surface disease (OSD).

- **Pretreat:** treat OSD and repeat keratometric measurements until stable.
- **Promote:** healthy wound healing by understanding OSD and surgical impacts on the cornea.
- **Provide:** stable optical interface and optical transparency when possible.
- **Prevent:** intraoperative visualization interference from opacities and dystrophies.

Table 2.1 Tear film and corneal disorders

Anterior visual components	Optical impacts	Surgical impacts	Surgical strategies
Tear film	HOA, visual fluctuations, light scatter, subjective complaints: glare, eye fatigue	Hazy view	Stabilize the tear film, heal the SPK preoperatively and postoperatively
Hyperosmolarity with chronic dry eye disease	Keratometric abnormalities Errors in astigmatism axis and magnitude (see ▶ Fig. 2.1)	• IOL calculation errors • Astigmatic axis and power errors	• Treat any suspected OSD • Repeat measurements until stable
Anterior basement membrane dystrophy	Topographic irregularities Multiple subjective optical aberrations	Inaccurate corneal power determination	Remove diseased epithelium and basement membrane preoperatively
Postrefractive surgery	Central corneal flatness underestimated by topography	Postcataract hyperopic refraction	• Advanced IOL calculation formulae • ORA intra-op measurements
Irregular corneal astigmatism	• HOA • Loss of BCVA	Corneal power	Stabilize degenerative conditions (e.g., cross-linking for keratoconus)
Corneal opacities	Light pathway interference	Visualization intra-op	• Pretreat if possible (e.g., femtolamellar excisions) • Chandelier retroillumination; oblique light illumination technique
Endothelial disease	Due to edema in late stages	Corneal edema intra-op	DSAEK or DMAEK

Abbreviations: BCVA, best-corrected visual acuity; DMAEK, Descemet's membrane automated endothelial keratoplasty; DSAEK, Descemet's stripping automated endothelial keratoplasty; HOA, higher order aberrations; intra-op: intraoperative; IOL, intraocular lens; OSD: ocular surface disorder; SPK, superficial punctate keratitis.

References

[1] The TFOS Dry Eye Workshop II. Ocul Surf. 2017(3):1–649

[2] Trattler WB, Majmudar PA, Donnenfeld ED, McDonald MB, Stonecipher KG, Goldberg DF. The Prospective Health Assessment of Cataract Patients' Ocular Surface (PHACO) study: the effect of dry eye. Clin Ophthalmol. 2017; 11:1423–1430

[3] Koh S. Mechanisms of visual disturbance in dry eye. Cornea. 2016; 35 suppl 1:S83–S88

[4] Epitropoulos AT, Matossian C, Berdy GJ, Malhotra RP, Potvin R. Effect of tear osmolarity on repeatability of keratometry for cataract surgery planning. J Cataract Refract Surg. 2015; 41(8):1672–1677

[5] Iaccheri B, Torroni G, Cagini C, et al. Corneal confocal scanning laser microscopy in patients with dry eye disease treated with topical cyclosporine. Eye (Lond). 2017; 31(5): 788–794

[6] McDonnel P, Pflugfelder S, Schiffman R, et al. Progression of Ocular Findings (PROOF) study of the natural history of dry eye: study design and baseline patient characteristics. IOVS. 2013; 54:4338

[7] Habeeb SY, Varma DK, Ahmed II. Oblique illumination and trypan blue to enhance visualization through corneal scars in cataract surgery. Can J Ophthalmol. 2011; 46(6):555–556

[8] Farjo AA, Meyer RF, Farjo QA. Phacoemulsification in eyes with corneal opacification. J Cataract Refract Surg. 2003; 29(2):242–245

[9] Nishimura A, Kobayashi A, PhD, et al. Endoillumination-assisted cataract surgery in a patient with corneal opacity. J Cataract Refract Surg. 2003; 29(12):2277–2280

3 Postrefractive Intraocular Lens Power Calculation: Choosing the Right Nomogram

Aazim A. Siddiqui and Uday Devgan

Abstract

Since the advent of refractive procedures in the late 20th century, a growing number of patients have undergone these procedures to enhance their vision and social outlook. As these patients grow older and develop cataracts, they require a surgical procedure to remove the opacified lens and implant an intraocular lens (IOL). Given the vastly satisfactory outcomes of their refractive surgery, these patients understandably maintain high expectations from their subsequent cataract surgery. Although the process of choosing an appropriate IOL remains a challenging task in virgin eyes, the task is even more complex in postrefractive eyes. Ironically, the therapeutic effects of refractive surgery make the outcome of IOL calculations for an eventual cataract surgery relatively suboptimal. Most modern IOL formulae and instruments were devised prior to the popularity of refractive surgery. Thus, they provide a high level of accuracy for eyes with physiologic corneas, but not so for ones that have undergone corneal flattening or steepening effects of myopic or hyperopic refractive surgery, respectively. These corneal changes result in inaccurate measurement and calculation of two important components of modern IOL formulae: corneal power and estimated lens position. Consequently, experts in the field have developed a multitude of various methods, formulae, and devices to address these challenges. Further, newer and more sophisticated methodologies and devices are forthcoming, which may result in more precise calculations and measurements. Therefore, it becomes important to understand and consider these methods carefully in combination with clinical judgment to achieve improved refractive outcomes.

Keywords: cataract, cataract surgery, postrefractive cataract surgery, intraocular lens, intraocular lens calculations, intraocular lens formula, laser-assisted in situ keratomileusis, photorefractive keratectomy, LASIK, PRK

3.1 Introduction

Every year, approximately a million patients in the United States choose to undergo some form of corneal refractive surgery to correct their vision.[1] This growing patient population will subsequently develop a cataract with age and have high expectations from their cataract surgery refractive outcomes like those of their previous refractive procedures. Advances in technology, instrumentation, and surgical technique have led to significant improvement in cataract procedures. However, compared to the results of refractive surgery, cataract surgery outcomes in these patients are relatively suboptimal.[2] A major reason for this disparity is due to the inadequate accuracy of intraocular lens (IOL) power calculation formulae in postrefractive eyes. Given the rising number of patients with a history of refractive surgery and their high expectations, calculating accurate IOL power for postrefractive eyes is of considerable importance.

Many different forms of refractive procedures exist that are based on a variation of approach, instrumentation, and anatomy. Procedures involving myopic correction with excimer laser treatment (i.e., photorefractive keratectomy [PRK], laser in situ keratomileusis [LASIK]) are of most interest as a growing number of patients have undergone this procedure in the previous few decades.

After the advent and Food and Drug Administration (FDA) approval of myopic LASIK in the late 1990s, it was found that accurate IOL power calculation prior to cataract surgery is more challenging in eyes that underwent refractive surgery than those that did not.[3,4] Cataract surgeries in patients with a history of these refractive procedures may lead to an undesirable hyperopic refractive result. Conversely, cataract surgery in patients with a history of hyperopic LASIK may lead to an undesirable myopic refractive shift. These risks are due to the changes to the corneal surface that take place as part of refractive surgery, which affect the process of accurate IOL calculations.

Experts in the field have described a variety of methodologies and approaches to minimize the errors in postrefractive IOL calculations.[5,6,7] Despite the continued improvement in outcomes of these patients, there is lack of a single, perfect solution to this problem, as demonstrated by the existence of a plethora of formulae, devices, and potential solutions.[8]

3.2 Origins of Error

Modern IOL formulae have evolved over the years and have become extremely sophisticated and accurate in their ability to calculate lens power. These theoretical and regression formulae were mostly developed prior to the advancement of refractive surgery. Thus, these formulae are accurate for physiologic corneas but not so for nonphysiologic corneas such as those altered by refractive surgery.

Third-generation IOL formulae such as Hoffer Q, Holladay I, and Sanders–Retzlaff–Kraff (SRK)/T rely on two main variables: axial length and corneal power.[6] These two variables are crucial components in the calculation of vergence and estimation of the postoperative lens position (i.e., estimated lens position [ELP] or anterior chamber depth [ACD]). As subsequent generations of IOL formulae have been developed, more variables have been introduced in formulae such as Holladay II, Barrett, and Haigis to further refine the lens power calculation. However, axial length and corneal power remain the two primary variables in the modern IOL formulae.

Modern IOL formulae and instruments are based on certain assumptions about the optical and anatomical characteristics of a virgin cornea. However, following most corneal refractive procedures, these assumptions are invalidated. Thus, when standard IOL formulae and biometric instruments are used in these eyes, a significant "refractive surprise" may be encountered after cataract surgery.

There are two main sources of error that a surgeon will encounter when attempting IOL calculations for postrefractive eyes: (1) the imprecise measurement of the true corneal power after refractive surgery[9,10] and (2) the inaccurate predictability of the ELP by the third- and fourth-generation IOL formulae.[11]

3.2.1 Keratometric Error

The refractive power of the cornea is one of the two most important variables in IOL calculations.[5] It is the most obvious source of error in performing IOL calculations in postrefractive eyes. This is due to the changes to the cornea that occur as a result of refractive surgery. These changes can vary from being a dramatic resurfacing to an alteration of refractive index of the cornea.[12,13]

Standard manual keratometry, automated keratometry, and topography instruments for virgin eyes are not suitable for the measurement of

postrefractive eyes[4,14] due to the surgical manipulation of the anterior cornea. As only the anterior surface of the cornea is impacted, this affects the refractive relationship between the anterior and posterior surface of the cornea. Not only are standard keratometers unable to account for the changes to the anterior surface of the cornea, but also they are unable to directly measure the posterior corneal power.

Measuring the Anterior Cornea

Traditional keratometry instruments measure the corneal power at four points of a paracentral 2.5- to 3.2-mm ring. These devices work on the assumption that a cornea is a spherocylindrical surface. Indeed, in a virgin eye, that holds true, as the central 2- to 3-mm area of the cornea is approximately spherical. In the postrefractive eye, however, the spherical nature of the central cornea is affected due to surgical manipulation (▶ Fig. 3.1).[15,16] Thus, these devices ignore flatter or steeper more central regions after myopic or hyperopic refractive surgery, respectively.[10] Such measurement technique will not provide an accurate measurement of the central flattening or steepening of the anterior cornea that occurs

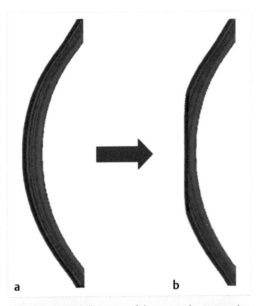

Fig. 3.1 Anterior flattening of the cornea due to myopic refractive surgery. Cross-sectional graphical renderings are shown in the (a) axial plane of a physiologic cornea and (b) anteriorly flattened central cornea due to myopic refractive surgery. It is important to note that the posterior cornea remains unaffected.

with myopic or hyperopic laser refractive surgery, respectively.[17]

Measuring the Posterior Cornea

A standard keratometer or topographer measures the corneal power (P) value by deriving it from the measured radius of curvature of the anterior corneal surface (r) and the "effective" index of refraction (n) according to the following formula:

$$P = (n - 1)/r.$$

However, these keratometers and topographers are unable to directly measure the radius of curvature of the posterior cornea (i.e., power of the posterior cornea). For virgin eyes, most keratometers and topographers compensate for the negative power of the posterior cornea by assuming that the radius of curvature of the posterior surface of the cornea is 1.2 mm less than the anterior curvature.[18] Based on Gullstrand's model eye,[19] a modified index of refraction of 1.3375 is used as opposed to 1.3760 of the cornea itself. However, refractive surgery, by causing a decrease or increase of anterior corneal curvature, alters and invalidates the anterior-to-posterior cornea relationship (▶ Fig. 3.1). Thus, the index of refraction (1.3375) used by standard keratometers would be invalid and result in measurement of unreliable corneal power values.[12,20,21]

3.2.2 Estimated Lens Position Error

The ELP is a calculated prediction of the postoperative distance between the optical center of the implanted IOL and the anterior surface of the cornea. Thus, it cannot be physically measured preoperatively. The incorrect calculation of the ELP in third- and fourth-generation IOL formulae is further responsible for the inaccuracy of IOL power calculation in postrefractive eyes.[6] Newer generations of IOL formulae have sought to improve the ELP predictability by introducing additional measurable variables such as preoperative refraction, horizontal white-to-white distance, ACD, lens thickness, and patient age.[4]

The anterior cornea radius of curvature (i.e., corneal power) is closely related to the ELP predictability. After myopic refractive surgery, the cornea is flatter than before. This affects the calculation of the ELP using traditional IOL formulae as a more forward lens position is predicted. This overestimation of ELP results in calculation of an underpowered IOL. Implantation of an underpowered IOL will then result in more hyperopic refractive outcomes.[6] Conversely, after hyperopic refractive surgery, the cornea is steeper than before. In these eyes, an underestimation of the ELP occurs, which then results in calculation of an overpowered IOL. Implantation of such an IOL will result in more myopic refractive outcomes.[12,22]

3.2.3 Surgery-Specific Error

The result of using standard methods of keratometry in a patient with a history of myopic LASIK or PRK refractive surgery would be an overestimation of the true corneal power.[23] This overestimation, thus, leads to more hyperopic results than intended after cataract surgery as a lower powered lens is calculated by IOL formulae.

Conversely, hyperopic refractive surgery such as LASIK and conductive keratoplasty (CK) will cause the keratometric process to result in an underestimation of the corneal power. As the central cornea is now steeper, standard methods of keratometry are unable to appropriately measure the now steeper cornea.[22] The effects of this underestimation yield an IOL power higher than intended and thus results in more myopic refractive outcomes after cataract surgery.[11,24,25]

Unlike the effects of LASIK and PRK, radial keratotomy affects both the anterior and posterior corneal surfaces. This may more closely preserve the anterior–posterior corneal relationship.[16] It could also cause a more severe overestimation as the cornea undergoes greater central-than-paracentral flattening.[26,27] Due to the variability of refractive change in the anterior and posterior cornea, refractive outcomes after cataract surgery in patients with a history of radial keratotomy are less predictable.[15]

3.3 Solutions to Postrefractive IOL Calculations

There is a plethora of solutions available to address the problems that exist with IOL calculations in patients with a history of refractive surgery (▶ Table 3.1). The proposed methods can be organized by those that require prerefractive "historical" data or not, and further by those that require topographic measurements or not.

3.3.1 Historical Data Methods

The current "gold standard" for IOL calculations in postrefractive eyes is to rely on the biometric and

Table 3.1 Intraocular lens calculation methods for postrefractive eyes

Historical data methods		Nonhistorical data methods	
Without topography	*With topography*	*Without topography*	*With topography*
Clinical history	Adjusted EffRP	Contact lens over-refraction	Maloney
Feiz–Mannis	Adjusted Atlas 9000 (4-mm zone)	Shammas	BESSt formula
Corneal bypass	Adjusted Atlas ring values	Haigis-L formula	Use of posterior corneal measurement devices
Aramberri double-K	Adjusted ACCP/APP	Intraoperative refraction	
Masket		Galilei TCP	
Modified Masket		Potvin–Hill Pentacam	
		Wang–Koch–Maloney	
		OCT based	

Abbreviations: ACCP, average central corneal power; APP, average pupil power; EffRP, effective refractive power; OCT, optical coherence tomography; TCP, total corneal power.

refractive data prior to the refractive surgery. These data include the prerefractive corneal power (K_{pre}), manifest refraction (MR), and surgically induced refractive change (RC) in manifest refraction. However, care must be taken to ensure that these data are accurate and acquired using calibrated instruments. If any data are incorrect, it may result in substantial discrepancy in the IOL power calculation.

Methods Using Historical Data without Topography

If a patient's prerefractive surgery information is known, it can allow the surgeon to use certain methods without topographic measurements to calculate IOL power in postrefractive eyes.

Clinical History Method

Originally introduced by Jack Holladay in 1989, the "clinical history" method was one of the first to address the challenges of IOL calculations in post-refractive eyes[28] and it remained the "gold standard" for several years.[12] It is based on the simple assumption that the change in refraction that an eye undergoes with refractive surgery is solely due to the corneal flattening effect of the surgery.

If preoperative keratometry is known for a given patient, then the postoperative keratometry can be estimated. This is done by a simple subtraction of the change in spherical equivalence due to refractive surgery from the preoperative corneal power. In most instances, this is a reasonable method, which provides accurate results. However, a few

factors are important to consider with this methodology as they may affect the accuracy and viability[12,28]:
- Preoperative data are not always available, in which case this method would not be a choice.
- Postoperative refraction may not necessarily be reliable or stable.
- With the development of cataract, an eye may also experience myopic shift.

Feiz–Mannis Method

The Feiz–Mannis method[24,26] adds a LASIK-induced correction factor to the IOL power that is calculated using the pre-LASIK corneal power and precataract surgery axial length. The eye is treated as if it has not undergone refractive surgery. A nomogram is also available for eyes where prerefractive keratometry is not available, but the refractive change done due to surgery is known.[12,25]

Corneal Bypass Method

The bypass method was described by Ladas et al[29] that takes the prerefractive corneal power and the refractive correction that occurs during the refractive surgery as target for emmetropia in a chosen formula.[30]

Aramberri's Double-K Method

Aramberri described a "double-K" method[5] by modifying the SRK/T formula, with which the pre-refractive surgery corneal power of around 43.00 diopter was used for the ELP calculation and the postrefractive corneal power was used for the vergence formula. This showed more accurate results compared to the clinical history method. Ladas et al described the corneal bypass method to generalize this approach to other third-generation formulae.[29] Aramberri's double-K provided a spreadsheet to calculate the ELP using the prerefractive corneal power with the SRK/T formula.[5,12]

Masket's Method

The Masket method[31] is based on a simple regression formula that uses corneal power values from IOL Master (Zeiss, Oberkochen, Germany). This approach was based on a total of 30 eyes that underwent either myopic or hyperopic refractive surgery. It modifies the IOL power calculated by the SRK/T formula with the known refractive change due to both myopic and hyperopic surgery as follows:

$$\text{IOL power adjustment} = (RC \times 0.326) + 0.101,$$

where RC is the refractive change induced by the surgery at the corneal plane.

Modified Masket Method

Others further modified the Masket method as follows[32]:

$$\text{IOL power adjustment} = (RC \times 0.4385) + 0.0295.$$

The Masket IOL power adjustment method can also be used after hyperopic in addition to myopic surgery.

Methods Using Historical Data with Topography

Several methods have also been proposed to calculate IOL power in postrefractive eyes with historical and topographical data. These methods use correction factors for ELP and topography for obtaining accurate postrefractive corneal power (K_{post}). The rationale for these methods is to reconcile the "new" proportional relationship between the anterior and posterior cornea.

Adjusted Effective Refractive Power Method

This method is a modification of the effective refractive power (EffRP) on the Holladay Diagnostic Summary of the EyeSys Corneal Analysis System (EyeSys Vision Inc., Houston, TX). The EffRP is the average refractive power of the central 3-mm cornea. This value is then adjusted by subtracting

0.15 diopter of power per diopter of RC induced at the corneal plane by refractive surgery[33,34]:

$$K_{post-myopic} = EffRP - (RC \times 0.15) - 0.05.$$

$$K_{post-hyperopic} = EffRP - (RC \times 0.162) - 0.279.$$

Wang et al[6,35] described a method of using these topographic measurements of corneal power (EffRPadj or Maloney method) in combination with a double-K approach.[5] Subsequent presentations by the authors have included more topographers and correction factors.[12]

Adjusted Atlas 9000 (4-mm zone) Method

This method is a modification of the 4-mm zone corneal power value from the Humphrey Atlas 9000 topographer (Zeiss) based on RC induced at the corneal plane by refractive surgery:

$$K_{post-myopic} = \text{Atlas 9000 } 4 - \text{mm zone} \\ - (0.162 \times RC) - 0.279.$$

Adjusted Atlas Ring Values Method

This method is a modification of the average corneal power of the 0-, 1-, 2-, and 3-mm ring values obtained from the Humphrey Atlas 9000 or 992–995 series topographer (Zeiss) based on RC induced at the corneal plane by refractive surgery. This adjustment can be performed for both postmyopic and posthyperopic eyes:

$$K_{post-myopic} = \text{Atlas Ring Values} - (RC \times 0.2).$$

$$K_{post-hyperopic} = \text{Atlas Ring Values} - (RC \times 0.19) \\ - 0.396.$$

Adjusted Average Central Corneal Power Method

This method is a modification of the average central corneal power (ACCP) of Placido rings over the central 3-mm cornea obtained from the Tomey Topography Modeling System (Tomey USA, Phoenix, AZ) or average pupil power (APP) from OPD-Scan III (Nidek Co., Ltd., Maehama, Japan). This modification is based on the RC at the corneal plane by refractive surgery:

$$K_{post-myopic} = \text{ACCP or APP} - (RC \times 0.16).$$

3.3.2 Nonhistorical Data Methods

Several approaches to IOL calculations in postrefractive eyes have been described when biometric and refractive data prior to the refractive surgery are unavailable. These methods rely on algorithms that modify the postrefractive corneal power values (K_{post}) to estimate the prerefractive corneal power values (K_{pre}).

Methods without Using Historical Data and Topography

If a patient's prerefractive surgery information is not known, one may choose to use certain methods without topographic measurements to calculate IOL power in postrefractive eyes.

Contact Lens Method

The contact lens over-refraction (OR) is one of the traditional methods that is rarely used in practice. In cases where prerefractive keratometric data are unavailable for a given patient, this method may be utilized.[18,36] A patient is given a contact lens of a known power and base. The resulting manifest refraction is then subtracted from the contact lens OR and then added to the base curve (BC) of the rigid contact lens and contact lens power (CLP) to obtain the postrefractive corneal power[4,12,37]:

$$K_{post} = BC + CLP + (OR - MR).$$

The disadvantages of this method include the unreliability of the MR due to the presence of the cataract and decreased best-corrected visual acuity (a patient must have at least 20/80 vision to be considered).[21]

Shammas' Method

Shammas et al described a regression-based method of adjusting measured postrefractive corneal power (K_{post}) to come up with an adjusted postrefractive corneal power (K_c) in order to estimate the prerefractive corneal power[38,39]:

$$K_c = (K_{post} \times 1.14) - 6.8.$$

Haigis-L Formula

Wolfgang Haigis developed a formula modification based on 40 eyes that requires no previous patient data. It is a regression approach based on the clinical history method that adjusts corneal power values as measured by the IOL Master device. Further, he arbitrarily adjusted the corneal power to achieve a small degree of myopia. Using these correction factors, an adjusted radius of curvature ($r_{adjusted}$) is calculated from the measured radius

of curvature ($r_{measured}$). This adjusted radius of curvature is then used as a variable in the fourth-generation Haigis IOL formula[40]:

$$r_{adjusted} = 331.5/(-5.1625 \times r_{measured} + 82.2603 - 0.35).$$

Intraoperative Refraction Method

There are methods that do not use IOL formulae altogether in order to calculate the IOL power for a postrefractive eye. One method is to take aphakic refractive measurements using an intraoperative aberrometer or a portable autorefractor. This technique helps determine the IOL power for emmetropia during cataract surgery. Measurements are taken after the removal of cataract and prior to implantation of the IOL. Aphakic refractive measurements can be taken immediately after cataract removal with the patient still in the operating room or 30 minutes after lens extraction with the patient in an examination room.[41] After the readings have been acquired, the IOL power is obtained by modifying the aphakic refraction (AR) with the lens A-constant (A) using an equation such as the one by Mackool[12,42]:

$$IOL\ power = (AR \times 1.75) + A - 118.4.$$

Galilei Total Corneal Power Method

Defined by Wang and Koch, this method is an adjustment to the total corneal power (TCP) obtained from the Galilei corneal topographer (Ziemer Ophthalmic Systems, Port, Switzerland) averaged over the central 4-mm cornea and calculated by ray tracing through anterior and posterior corneal surfaces using the Snell law:

$$K_{post} = TCP \times 1.0887 - 1.8348.$$

Potvin–Hill Pentacam Method

This method is an adjustment to the true net power (TNP) measured over the 4-mm central corneal zone using Pentacam Scheimpflug device (Oculus Inc., Wetzlar, Germany)[43]:

$$ACD\ not\ known \rightarrow K_{post} = 12.08 + 0.9 \times TNP - 0.282 \times axial\ length.$$

$$ACD\ known \rightarrow K_{post} = 11.19 + 0.951 \times TNP - 0.247 \times axial\ length - 0.588 \times ACD.$$

Wang–Koch–Maloney Method

This method calculates postrefractive corneal power by converting the average corneal power from Humphrey Atlas topographer's 0-, 1-, 2-, and 3-mm zones to anterior corneal power[44]:

$$K_{post} = (Atlas\ 0\ to\ 3\ mm\ zone\ average\ \times .114) - 5.59.$$

Optical Coherence Tomography Based Method

This method requires acquisition of the net corneal power, posterior corneal power, and central corneal thickness from RTVue or RTVue-XR (Optovue Inc., Fremont, CA) device. It also requires axial length and ACD from IOL Master. These parameters are then used as input for the optical coherence tomography (OCT) based IOL formula as outlined by Huang et al.[45]

Methods Using Topography without Historical Data

If a patient's prerefractive surgery information is not known, one may choose to use certain methods using solely topographic measurements to calculate IOL power in postrefractive eyes. These methods use the measured postrefractive corneal power (K_{post}) to come up with an adjusted postrefractive corneal power (K_c).

Maloney Method

The Maloney method involves modifying the central corneal power from a topographic map using the following formula[46]:

$$K_c = (K_{post}\ /1.114) - 4.90\ diopter.$$

Wang et al further modified this correction by subtracting a greater value than the original 4.90 diopter as proposed by Maloney[46]:

$$K_c = (K_{post}\ /1.114) - 6.10\ diopter.$$

BESSt (Gaussian) Formula

The Borasio Edmondo Smith and Stevens (BESSt) formula was devised by Borasio et al[44] and is based on Gaussian optics principles that use the anterior and posterior corneal powers from the Pentacam device to estimate postrefractive corneal power:

$$F_{tot} = F_{ant} + F_{post} - (d\ /n) \times (F_{ant} \times F_{post}),$$

where d is the corneal thickness in microns, n is the corneal refractive index, and F_{tot}, F_{ant}, and F_{post} are the total, anterior, and posterior corneal powers in diopters, respectively.

Posterior Corneal Power Measurement

Most standard topographers measure only the anterior corneal power and indirectly account for the posterior corneal power. However, various devices have also been introduced that attempt to measure the posterior corneal power directly in postrefractive eyes. These include the scanning slit topographers that measure both the anterior and posterior corneal powers. Orbscan II (Bausch & Lomb, Rochester, NY) is an example of a topographer that measures the true corneal power by determining power of the central corneal zone as well as the posterior corneal surface. Based on the type of surgery the patient has undergone, a more optimal diameter zone can be chosen based on findings in the literature. For example, the optimal diameter zone of 4.50 and 5.00 mm has been found to be more appropriate for eyes that undergone LASIK and radial keratectomy surgeries, respectively.[47] The Oculus Pentacam is a rotating Scheimpflug camera anterior segment imaging system that is another example of a device that can measure both the anterior and posterior corneal powers.[12,44] Galilei Dual Scheimpflug Analyzer (Ziemer Ophthalmic Systems) is an example of another corneal topographer which measures both the anterior and posterior corneal surfaces and corneal thickness by combining dual-channel Scheimpflug cameras with an integrated Placido disc to measure both anterior and posterior corneal surfaces and corneal thickness.[48]

3.4 Conclusion

Indeed, there exist a wide variety of solutions for each given scenario in order to achieve the best IOL calculation outcomes in postrefractive cataract surgery. Standard IOL formulae and measurement devices are inadequate when accounting for important parameters that represent a postrefractive eye. There is no single, perfect solution that would be applicable to all situations.

There is a paucity of large clinical studies that provide appropriate conclusions regarding the ideal solution in a particular eye. Based on the availability of a patient's stable and reliable prior refractive and biometric information, either the clinical history method or one of the "nonhistorical" data regression methods such as Shammas and Haigis-L can be used. In the absence of prerefractive data, a surgeon could also opt for one of the methods that rely on adjusting postrefractive corneal power measured using standard keratometers and topographers. A surgeon may choose to use multiple methods and select the flattest or steepest keratometric values in the case of a postmyopic or posthyperopic patient, respectively.

There is also a continuing development of advanced topographic instruments that are able to provide accurate measurements of both the anterior and posterior corneal power values after refractive surgery. These devices may help overcome many of the deficiencies that exist in current methods of performing these calculations. More studies are needed to draw further conclusions about the latest instruments and methods.

Finally, newer generations of IOL formulae are forthcoming that use complex mathematical techniques of formula hybridization in combination with artificial intelligence. These solutions may further refine the accuracy and simplify the process of postrefractive IOL calculations.

The task of picking the most appropriate methodology to perform IOL power calculations in postrefractive eyes remains a challenge. However, the use of appropriate methods, formulae, devices, and clinical decision-making is the pathway to improved accuracy in postrefractive cataract surgery outcomes.

3.5 Key Pearls

- A growing number of patients with a history of postrefractive surgery will subsequently undergo cataract surgery.
- IOL calculation is a major cause for suboptimal outcomes of cataract surgery in postrefractive eyes.
- Standard IOL formulae and biometric devices are unable to accurately account for the changes to the eye due to refractive surgery.
- A plethora of various formulae and solutions have been proposed by experts in the field to improve accuracy of lens calculations in postrefractive eyes.
- A surgeon must use clinical judgment in combination with the available patient data and topographic measurements to choose the most appropriate IOL calculation methodology.
- Newer generation of IOL formulae and more advanced corneal topographers are emerging, which may help improve accuracy of IOL calculations in postrefractive eyes.

References

[1] Helzner J. Can you revive your refractive surgery practice? Ophthalmol Manag. September 2010. https://www.ophthalmologymanagement.com/issues/2010/september-2010/can-you-revive-your-refractive-surgery-practice

[2] McCarthy M, Gavanski GM, Paton KE, Holland SP. Intraocular lens power calculations after myopic laser refractive surgery: a comparison of methods in 173 eyes. Ophthalmology. 2011; 118(5):940–944

[3] Seitz B, Langenbucher A, Nguyen NX, Kus MM, Küchle M. Underestimation of intraocular lens power for cataract surgery after myopic photorefractive keratectomy. Ophthalmology. 1999; 106(4):693–702

[4] Hamilton DR, Hardten DR. Cataract surgery in patients with prior refractive surgery. Curr Opin Ophthalmol. 2003; 14(1): 44–53

[5] Aramberri J. Intraocular lens power calculation after corneal refractive surgery: double-K method. J Cataract Refract Surg. 2003; 29(11):2063–2068

[6] Koch DD, Wang L. Calculating IOL power in eyes that have had refractive surgery. J Cataract Refract Surg. 2003; 29(11): 2039–2042

[7] Abdelghany AA, Alio JL. Surgical options for correction of refractive error following cataract surgery. Eye Vis (Lond). 2014; 1:2

[8] Skiadaresi E, McAlinden C, Pesudovs K, Polizzi S, Khadka J, Ravalico G. Subjective quality of vision before and after cataract surgery. Arch Ophthalmol. 2012; 130(11): 1377–1382

[9] Koch DD, Liu JF, Hyde LL, Rock RL, Emery JM. Refractive complications of cataract surgery after radial keratotomy. Am J Ophthalmol. 1989; 108(6):676–682

[10] Seitz B, Langenbucher A. Intraocular lens power calculation in eyes after corneal refractive surgery. J Refract Surg. 2000; 16(3):349–361

[11] Wang L, Jackson DW, Koch DD. Methods of estimating corneal refractive power after hyperopic laser in situ keratomileusis. J Cataract Refract Surg. 2002; 28(6):954–961

[12] Kalyani SD, Kim A, Ladas JG. Intraocular lens power calculation after corneal refractive surgery. Curr Opin Ophthalmol. 2008; 19(4):357–362

[13] Patel S, Alió JL, Pérez-Santonja JJ. Refractive index change in bovine and human corneal stroma before and after lasik: a study of untreated and re-treated corneas implicating stromal hydration. Invest Ophthalmol Vis Sci. 2004; 45(10): 3523–3530

[14] Holladay JT. Measurements. In: Yanoff M, Duker JS, eds. Ophthalmology. 2nd ed. St Louis, MO: Mosby; 2004:287–292

[15] Jonna G, Channa P. Updated practical intraocular lens power calculation after refractive surgery. Curr Opin Ophthalmol. 2013; 24(4):275–280

[16] Wang L. Intraocular lens power calculations in eyes with prior corneal refractive surgery. J Clin Exp Ophthalmol. 2012; 3(8)

[17] Arrowsmith PN, Marks RG. Visual, refractive, and keratometric results of radial keratotomy. Five-year follow-up. Arch Ophthalmol. 1989; 107(4):506–511

[18] Holladay JT. Cataract surgery in patients with previous keratorefractive surgery (RK, PRK, and LASIK). Ophthalmol Pract. 1997; 15(6):238–244

[19] Olsen T. On the calculation of power from curvature of the cornea. Br J Ophthalmol. 1986; 70(2):152–154

[20] Norrby S. Pentacam keratometry and IOL power calculation. J Cataract Refract Surg. 2008; 34(1):3–, author reply 4

[21] Haigis W. Corneal power after refractive surgery for myopia: contact lens method. J Cataract Refract Surg. 2003; 29(7): 1397–1411

[22] Chokshi AR, Latkany RA, Speaker MG, Yu G. Intraocular lens calculations after hyperopic refractive surgery. Ophthalmology. 2007; 114(11):2044–2049

[23] Koch DD. Cataract surgery following refractive surgery. Am Acad Ophthalmol Focal Points. 2001; 19:1–7

[24] Feiz V, Mannis MJ, Garcia-Ferrer F, et al. Intraocular lens power calculation after laser in situ keratomileusis for myopia and hyperopia: a standardized approach. Cornea. 2001; 20(8):792–797

[25] Feiz V, Moshirfar M, Mannis MJ, et al. Nomogram-based intraocular lens power adjustment after myopic photorefractive keratectomy and LASIK: a new approach. Ophthalmology. 2005; 112(8):1381–1387

[26] Feiz V, Mannis MJ. Intraocular lens power calculation after corneal refractive surgery. Curr Opin Ophthalmol. 2004; 15 (4):342–349

[27] Hanna KD, Jouve FE, Waring GO, III. Preliminary computer simulation of the effects of radial keratotomy. Arch Ophthalmol. 1989; 107(6):911–918

[28] Latkany RA, Chokshi AR, Speaker MG, Abramson J, Soloway BD, Yu G. Intraocular lens calculations after refractive surgery. J Cataract Refract Surg. 2005; 31(3):562–570

[29] Ladas JG, Stark WJ. Calculating IOL power after refractive surgery. J Cataract Refract Surg. 2004; 30(12):2458–, author reply 2458–2459

[30] Walter KA, Gagnon MR, Hoopes PC, Jr, Dickinson PJ. Accurate intraocular lens power calculation after myopic laser in situ keratomileusis, bypassing corneal power. J Cataract Refract Surg. 2006; 32(3):425–429

[31] Masket S, Masket SE. Simple regression formula for intraocular lens power adjustment in eyes requiring cataract surgery after excimer laser photoablation. J Cataract Refract Surg. 2006; 32(3):430–434

[32] Hill WE. IOL power calculations following keratorefractive surgery. Presentation at: Cornea Day of the Annual Meeting of the American Society of Cataract and Refractive Surgery; San Francisco, CA, March 17, 2006

[33] Holladay JT. Corneal topography using the Holladay diagnostic summary. J Cataract Refract Surg. 1997; 23(2):209–221

[34] Hamed AM, Wang L, Misra M, Koch DD. A comparative analysis of five methods of determining corneal refractive power in eyes that have undergone myopic laser in situ keratomileusis. Ophthalmology. 2002; 109(4):651–658

[35] Wang L, Booth MA, Koch DD. Comparison of intraocular lens power calculation methods in eyes that have undergone laser-assisted in-situ keratomileusis. Trans Am Ophthalmol Soc. 2004; 102:189–196, discussion 196–197

[36] Zeh WG, Koch DD. Comparison of contact lens overrefraction and standard keratometry for measuring corneal curvature in eyes with lenticular opacity. J Cataract Refract Surg. 1999; 25(7):898–903

[37] Argento C, Cosentino MJ, Badoza D. Intraocular lens power calculation after refractive surgery. J Cataract Refract Surg. 2003; 29(7):1346–1351

[38] Shammas HJ, Shammas MC. No-history method of intraocular lens power calculation for cataract surgery after myopic laser in situ keratomileusis. J Cataract Refract Surg. 2007; 33 (1):31–36

[39] Shammas HJ, Shammas MC, Garabet A, Kim JH, Shammas A, LaBree L. Correcting the corneal power measurements for intraocular lens power calculations after myopic laser in situ keratomileusis. Am J Ophthalmol. 2003; 136(3):426–432

[40] Haigis W. Intraocular lens calculation after refractive surgery for myopia: Haigis-L formula. J Cataract Refract Surg. 2008; 34(10):1658–1663

[41] Ianchulev T, Salz J, Hoffer K, Albini T, Hsu H, Labree L. Intraoperative optical refractive biometry for intraocular lens power estimation without axial length and keratometry measurements. J Cataract Refract Surg. 2005; 31 (8):1530–1536

[42] Mackool RJ, Ko W, Mackool R. Intraocular lens power calculation after laser in situ keratomileusis: aphakic refraction technique. J Cataract Refract Surg. 2006; 32(3):435–437

[43] Potvin R, Hill W. New algorithm for intraocular lens power calculations after myopic laser in situ keratomileusis based on rotating Scheimpflug camera data. J Cataract Refract Surg. 2015; 41(2):339–347

[44] Borasio E, Stevens J, Smith GT. Estimation of true corneal power after keratorefractive surgery in eyes requiring cataract surgery: BESSt formula. J Cataract Refract Surg. 2006; 32(12):2004–2014

[45] Huang D, Tang M, Wang L, et al. Optical coherence tomography-based corneal power measurement and intraocular lens power calculation following laser vision correction (an American Ophthalmological Society thesis). Trans Am Ophthalmol Soc. 2013; 111:34–68

[46] Wang L, Booth MA, Koch DD. Comparison of intraocular lens power calculation methods in eyes that have undergone LASIK. Ophthalmology. 2004; 111(10):1825–1831

[47] Qazi MA, Cua IY, Roberts CJ, Pepose JS. Determining corneal power using Orbscan II videokeratography for intraocular lens calculation after excimer laser surgery for myopia. J Cataract Refract Surg. 2007; 33(1):21–30

[48] Wang L, Mahmoud AM, Anderson BL, Koch DD, Roberts CJ. Total corneal power estimation: ray tracing method versus gaussian optics formula. Invest Ophthalmol Vis Sci. 2011; 52 (3):1716–1722

4 Residual Refractive Error

Lisa Y. Chen and Edward E. Manche

Abstract

This chapter discusses the causes of residual refractive error after cataract surgery and the surgical strategies that can be utilized by the modern-day ophthalmologist to manage and correct this unintended pseudophakic ametropia.

Keywords: residual refractive error, LASIK, PRK, arcuate keratotomy, IOL exchange, piggyback IOL, toric IOL, light-adjustable IOL

4.1 Residual Refractive Error

Continued research efforts to further advance and refine technologies and techniques within cataract surgery have significantly optimized postoperative refractive outcomes over time. However, even in the hands of the most experienced and skilled surgeon, a subset of patients may still be left with residual refractive error that negatively affects vision.[1] Fortunately, there is currently an unprecedented number of strategies available for managing residual refractive error, each of which can yield favorable results when implemented appropriately.

4.2 Causes of Residual Refractive Error after Cataract Surgery

Prior to pursuing any treatment, it is critical for the surgeon to first determine the cause of refractive surprise so that the most appropriate management can be selected. In general, pseudophakic residual refractive error may be the result of preoperative, intraoperative, and/or postoperative causes. Preoperative causes include biometry errors leading to inaccurate axial length or keratometry readings, which subsequently affect the calculation of intraocular lens (IOL) power.[2] Similarly, failure to recognize corneal pathology or elicit a history of prior keratorefractive surgery will lead to inaccurate topographic and keratometric measurements. Intraoperative causes include incorrect positioning of the IOL, misalignment of a toric IOL, or, more uncommonly, inadvertent selection of the incorrect IOL power. Postoperatively,

changes in the final IOL position can occur during the healing process due to capsular bag fibrosis.

4.3 Management of Residual Refractive Error after Cataract Surgery

Once the cause of refractive error has been determined, an individualized treatment plan can be tailored to meet the needs of the particular patient. Initially, conservative measures such as the use of spectacles or contact lenses should be attempted. For those patients who cannot or will not tolerate such noninvasive methods, surgical correction must be considered. Surgical strategies for the correction of residual refractive error can be thought of in two general categories: (1) cornea-based approaches and (2) lens-based approaches.

4.3.1 Cornea-Based Approaches

Keratorefractive Surgery

Keratorefractive approaches for correcting pseudophakic ametropia include laser in situ keratomileusis (LASIK) and photorefractive keratectomy (PRK). Both of these procedures have been extensively studied for their use in the correction of a wide range of refractive errors and have demonstrated excellent safety, efficacy, and predictability.[3] Laser refractive surgery not only avoids additional intraocular surgery and its inherent associated risks, but also appears to provide better accuracy when compared to IOL exchange or piggyback lens techniques. Specifically, LASIK-treated eyes have demonstrated superior predictability, with 93% of eyes achieving a final spherical equivalent (SE) within ±0.50 diopters of emmetropia, when compared to lens-based procedures.[4] Furthermore, LASIK is preferable in eyes that have previously undergone neodymium:YAG capsulotomy, where IOL exchange becomes more difficult with greater risk of intraoperative complications.[5] Refractive surgery does, however, have some disadvantages, including its limited ability to correct large spherical errors. In addition, the older patient population that undergoes cataract surgery may be more susceptible to tear film abnormalities that can develop after corneal ablative procedures.

Arcuate Keratotomy

In those patients whose ametropia is composed primarily of cylindrical error, arcuate keratotomy can be performed, either manually or with femtosecond technology, to correct this residual corneal astigmatism. In fact, a recent study found femtosecond laser-assisted arcuate keratotomy to be as effective as implantation of a toric IOL in correcting corneal astigmatism.[6]

4.3.2 Lens-Based Approaches

Intraocular Lens Exchange

Implantation of the incorrect IOL power and IOL dislocation/decentration are currently the two most commonly reported indications for IOL exchange after cataract surgery.[7] However, as multifocal IOLs become increasingly popular, patient dissatisfaction from resulting higher-order aberrations such as glare and halos is contributing to an ever-increasing proportion of IOL exchange cases. Nonetheless, given the risks associated with further intraocular surgery, it is preferable to reserve IOL exchange to patients who require large ametropic corrections or those with severe corneal disease prohibiting them from receiving keratorefractive surgery. In all cases, IOL exchange is best performed soon after the initial surgery when the original cataract wound can be reopened and capsular-IOL adhesions have not yet formed.

Piggyback Intraocular Lens Implantation

The piggyback technique that involves the implantation of a second IOL not only can be used to correct high levels of refractive error, but also offers several additional advantages, including improved ease of surgery, relative simplicity of IOL power calculation, and reversibility of the procedure. Furthermore, recent studies have shown piggyback IOLs to be more effective and accurate than IOL exchange, with a higher percentage of eyes achieving 20/20 uncorrected distance visual acuity or better (33 vs. 18%) and an SE within ±0.50 diopters of emmetropia (92 vs. 82%).[8] Potential drawbacks of this approach, however, include the risk of developing postoperative interlenticular opacities, pupillary block, pigment dispersion, or secondary glaucoma.

Rotation of a Toric Intraocular Lens

Refractive surprise after implantation of a toric IOL can occur due to a variety of reasons including preoperative measurement error, alignment error, IOL rotation, or surgically induced astigmatism. In cases of alignment error or IOL rotation, prompt diagnosis on the part of the surgeon is essential so that IOL orientation can be corrected in a timely manner postoperatively. However, it is important to remember that rotation of a toric IOL can also be an effective tool for treating residual refractive error in cases not involving axis misalignment, but rather corneal topographical changes over time, such as Salzmann's nodular degeneration or pterygium.[9]

Light-Adjustable Intraocular Lens

Another emerging lens-based technology is the light-adjustable IOL, which introduces the possibility of correcting postoperative ametropia in a noninvasive way. Using this technology, the refractive power of the IOL can be titrated using ultraviolet light based on the individual requirements of each patient postoperatively with correction of up to 2.0 diopters of refractive error (▶ Fig. 4.1). While this technology is still not yet commercially available in the United States, the results of preliminary international studies are quite promising, demonstrating excellent visual outcomes.[10]

4.4 Conclusion

Paralleling the advance of technology, patient's expectations after cataract surgery also continue to grow. As a result, ophthalmologists must be prepared to manage unintended pseudophakic ametropia. Familiarity with the causes and surgical treatment options for residual refractive error should therefore be an essential component of every modern-day cataract surgeon's armamentarium.

4.5 Key Pearls

- It is critical to first determine the cause of refractive surprise so that the most appropriate management can be selected.
- Keratorefractive surgery (LASIK or PRK) avoids the risks of intraocular surgery and yields more effective and predictable outcomes than lens-based procedures.

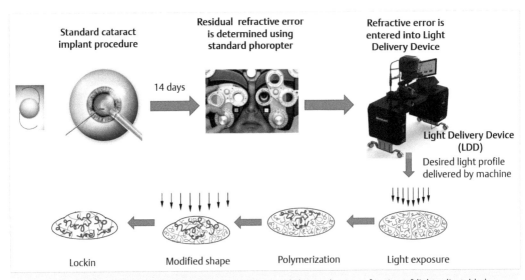

Fig. 4.1 Schematic depicting the timeline of implementation and the mechanism of action of light-adjustable lens technology. (Reproduced with permission of RxSight, Aliso Viejo, CA.)

- Piggyback IOLs are preferred to IOL exchange due to their ease of implantation and increased accuracy. However, both of these modalities should be reserved for cases of large spherical error or for those patients who are not candidates for corneal ablative treatments given the significant risks related to intraocular surgery.
- Arcuate keratotomy and toric IOL rotation are both tools that can effectively address residual corneal astigmatism.
- The light-adjustable IOL is an exciting emerging technology that may provide a noninvasive method to treat residual refractive error.

References

[1] Behndig A, Montan P, Stenevi U, Kugelberg M, Zetterström C, Lundström M. Aiming for emmetropia after cataract surgery: Swedish National Cataract Register study. J Cataract Refract Surg. 2012; 38(7):1181–1186

[2] Norrby S. Sources of error in intraocular lens power calculation. J Cataract Refract Surg. 2008; 34(3):368–376

[3] Schallhorn SC, Farjo AA, Huang D, et al. American Academy of Ophthalmology. Wavefront-guided LASIK for the correction of primary myopia and astigmatism a report by the American Academy of Ophthalmology. Ophthalmology. 2008; 115(7): 1249–1261

[4] Fernández-Buenaga R, Alió JL, Pérez Ardoy AL, Quesada AL, Pinilla-Cortés L, Barraquer RI. Resolving refractive error after cataract surgery: IOL exchange, piggyback lens, or LASIK. J Refract Surg. 2013; 29(10):676–683

[5] Jin GJ, Merkley KH, Crandall AS, Jones YJ. Laser in situ keratomileusis versus lens-based surgery for correcting residual refractive error after cataract surgery. J Cataract Refract Surg. 2008; 34(4):562–569

[6] Yoo A, Yun S, Kim JY, Kim MJ, Tchah H. Femtosecond laser-assisted arcuate keratotomy versus toric IOL implantation for correcting astigmatism. J Refract Surg. 2015; 31 (9):574–578

[7] Jones JJ, Jones YJ, Jin GJ. Indications and outcomes of intraocular lens exchange during a recent 5-year period. Am J Ophthalmol. 2014; 157(1):154–162.e1

[8] El Awady HE, Ghanem AA. Secondary piggyback implantation versus IOL exchange for symptomatic pseudophakic residual ametropia. Graefes Arch Clin Exp Ophthalmol. 2013; 251(7):1861–1866

[9] Lockwood JC, Randleman JB. Toric intraocular lens rotation to optimize refractive outcome despite appropriate intraoperative positioning. J Cataract Refract Surg. 2015; 41(4):878–883

[10] Villegas EA, Alcon E, Rubio E, Marín JM, Artal P. Refractive accuracy with light-adjustable intraocular lenses. J Cataract Refract Surg. 2014; 40(7):1075–84.e2

5 Posterior Corneal Astigmatism: Basics and Clinical Implications

Fernando Antonio Faria-Correia, José Carlos Ferreira Mendes, and Renato Ambrósio Jr.

Abstract

Until recently, corneal power calculations were based on the measurement of anterior corneal surface values taking into consideration a fixed posterior-to-anterior curvature ratio. Presence of posterior corneal astigmatism prompts to some of the unexpected surprises met after cataract surgery, as astigmatism is an important and often a visually significant optical aberration. This chapter discusses the importance of taking into consideration the posterior corneal power to optimize the postcataract surgery outcomes.

Keywords: posterior corneal astigmatism, corneal astigmatism, posterior corneal curvature, Scheimpflug imaging, simulated keratometry, with-the-rule astigmatism, against-the-rule astigmatism

5.1 Introduction

In the intraocular lens (IOL) power calculation setting, optical modeling has moved from thin-lens paraxial vergence calculations to thick-lens exact ray-tracing calculations. This is a direct consequence of improvements either in measuring devices or in calculation models and formulae. In the theoretical third-generation (i.e., Sanders–Retzlaff–Kraff [SRK]/T, Holladay 1, Hoffer Q, and Haigis) and fourth-generation (i.e., Holladay 2) formulae, cornea and IOL are thin lenses. Corneal power is calculated from the measured anterior radius using the keratometric index of refraction, 1.3375, which renders a figure that estimates the divergent or negative lens power effect of the unmeasured posterior surface. The accuracy of this method is based on two main implicit assumptions: anterior-to-posterior radius ratio fits the normal proportion (around 1.21) and posterior corneal toricity follows the anterior pattern with a constant and proportional magnitude.

Keratometers, both manual and automated, and front-surface reflection topographers have been providing these keratometric and simulated measurements for decades with acceptable clinical results in terms of spherical equivalent dioptric results in IOL surgery. However, the last 10 years have revealed the weaknesses of this method as clinical demand has risen with the emergence of refractive lens surgery, mostly related to the advent of multifocal and toric IOLs. New technologies, capable of measuring both the anterior and posterior corneal curvatures, have emerged, permitting the surgeon to target more precisely the total corneal power and astigmatism. With this development, there is a need to properly distinguish topography from tomography,[1] and Scheimpflug imaging, optical coherence tomography (OCT), and novel reflection-based devices are now competing for the position of the most accurate method to calculate these parameters. Knowledge of the effect of posterior corneal astigmatism (PCA) on the total has also allowed for the development to more accurate formulae.

5.2 Measuring the Posterior Corneal Astigmatism

In 2012, Koch and coworkers published a relevant work highlighting the contribution of PCA to total corneal astigmatism (TCA). In a retrospective study, 715 eyes from 435 patients were examined by Galilei dual Scheimpflug analyzer to calculate the TCA using a ray-tracing formula over the central 1 to 4 mm of the cornea. Mean magnitudes were as follows: TCA, +1.07 ± 0.71 diopters; anterior corneal astigmatism (ACA), +1.20 ± 0.79 diopters; corneal astigmatism from simulated keratometry (CA Sim K), +1.08 ± 0.71 diopters; and PCA, −0.30 ± 0.15 diopters. Vertical meridian was steeper in 86.8% of PCA, compared to 50.9% of ACA. Almost 5% had a vector difference of more than 0.50 diopters.[2] Later, Savini and coworkers published a similar work in eyes with more than 1.00 diopter of CA Sim K. PCA excessed 0.50 diopters in more than 55.4% of eyes. More than 16% presented a difference in astigmatism magnitude between TCA and CA Sim K higher than 0.50 diopters. Compared with TCA, CA Sim K overestimated with-the-rule (WTR) astigmatism (mean 0.22 ± 0.32 diopters); underestimated against-the-rule (ATR) astigmatism (mean 0.21 ± 0.26 diopters); and overestimated oblique astigmatism (mean 0.13 ± 0.37 diopters).[3]

5.3 Impact of Posterior Corneal Astigmatism on Toric Intraocular Lens Calculation

To validate their theory, Koch and coworkers tried to measure the impact of PCA in toric IOL calculation. Pre- and postoperative corneal astigmatism were assessed with different technology devices: automated keratometry, IOL Master, Lenstar LS900, Placido corneal topography, Atlas system, manual keratometer, Bausch and Lomb, Placido dual Scheimpflug analyzer, and Galilei. In vectorial analysis calculation, predicted error was not significant from zero only in Placido dual Scheimpflug analyzer. Corneal astigmatism was overestimated (0.5–0.6 diopters) in WTR by all devices and underestimated (0.2–0.3 diopters) in ATR by all devices, except the Placido dual Scheimpflug analyzer. The authors proposed a nomogram for toric IOL selection, based on preoperative corneal astigmatism, designated as "Baylor nomogram" (▶ Fig. 5.1).[4] In the Baylor nomogram, the planning in correction ATR astigmatism is toward an overcorrection, while the WTR astigmatism is calculated to be on target or undercorrected (▶ Table 5.1). In this estimation, the Baylor nomogram does not consider posterior cornea in determining the IOL axis alignment.[4]

The Pentacam HR, has also been used in similar works. Tonn and coworkers analyzed 3,818 healthy eyes comparing CA Sim K and TCA. The latter was measured in the 3-mm zone by ray tracing. Again, CA Sim K overestimated TCA in eyes with WTR astigmatism. CA Sim K could not predict TCA in eyes that did not have WTR astigmatism. In eyes with WTR anterior astigmatism, posterior astigmatism was vertical too in 97%; in eyes with ATR anterior astigmatism, 18% of the cases also presented a horizontally oriented posterior astigmatism.[5] ▶ Table 5.1 summarizes the results presented in the scientific studies that consider corneal astigmatism measurements.

5.4 Toric Intraocular Lens Calculation in Clinical Practice

Toric IOL calculations must consider the influence of the posterior cornea not relying just on the keratometric (Sim K) astigmatism anymore. This can be done using the measured posterior curvature in a thick-lens calculation model or using an algorithm that calculates that effect. The former method is particularly important in eyes that had previous corneal refractive surgery as the anterior/posterior astigmatism proportion has been changed, especially if any astigmatic correction was done in the anterior cornea. New-generation Scheimpflug and OCT tomographers can measure the TCA accurately (▶ Fig. 5.2). The Cassini (I-Optics, The Hague, The Netherlands) can measure the posterior cornea from LED (light-emitting diode) reflection analysis and calculates the total corneal power and astigmatism by ray tracing. Some of these devices incorporate IOL calculation software, which takes into account the different refractive effect of both corneal surfaces. Another

WTR Astigmatism	
Astigmatism diopter	Toric IOL
≤1.69	0 (PCRI if > 1.00)
1.70–2.19	T3
2.20–2.69	T4
2.70–3.19	T5

ATR Astigmatism	
Astigmatism diopter	Toric IOL
≤0.39	0
0.40–0.79	T3
0.80–1.29	T4
1.30–1.79	T5

Fig. 5.1 Baylor's nomogram. The nomogram targets up to 0.40 diopters of residual WTR astigmatism using an average 0.20-diopter WTR surgical-induced astigmatism. ATR, against the rule; IOL, intraocular lens; PCRI, peripheral corneal relaxing incision; WTR, with the rule.

Table 5.1 Summary of research articles

Authors (year)	Device studied	Study group	Findings
Koch et al[2] (2012)	Galilei (Ziemer, Port, Switzerland)	715 eyes (435 patients)	• The steep corneal meridian was aligned vertically (60–120 degrees) in 51.9% of eyes for the anterior surface and in 86.6% for the posterior surface. • With aging, the steep anterior corneal meridian tended to change from vertical to horizontal, while the steep posterior corneal meridian did not change. • The magnitude and alignment of total corneal astigmatism could not be accurately predicted from anterior corneal measurements. Therefore, ignoring posterior corneal astigmatism could cause unanticipated outcomes in eyes having toric intraocular implantation.
Savini et al[3] (2012)	Sirius (Costruzione Strumenti Oftalmici, Florence, Italy)	157 eyes (87 patients)	• In eyes with more than 1.00 diopter of keratometric astigmatism, posterior corneal astigmatism exceeded 0.50 diopter in a considerably higher percentage of cases (55.4%). • The effect of posterior corneal astigmatism on anterior corneal astigmatism was significantly higher in eyes with "with-the-rule" astigmatism (0.61 diopter) than in those with "against-the-rule" astigmatism (0.05 diopter). • On average, posterior corneal astigmatism compensated for "with-the-rule" keratometric astigmatism and increased "against-the-rule" keratometric astigmatism. However, in approximately 20% of cases, the opposite effect may occur.
Koch et al[4] (2013)	Automated keratometry, IOLMaster (Carl Zeiss, Jena, Germany), Lenstar LS900 (Haag-Streit, Koniz, Switzerland), Atlas corneal topographer (Carl Zeiss), manual keratometer (Bausch & Lomb Inc, Rochester, NY), and Galilei (Ziemer)	41 eyes (41 patients)	• "Baylor nomogram" for toric intraocular lens selection aims for a residual "with-the-rule" refractive astigmatism and accounts for the effect of "against-the rule" drift that occurs with aging. • In eyes with toric intraocular lens implantation, corneal astigmatism prediction errors with devices that measure anterior corneal astigmatism only, corneal astigmatism was overestimated (0.5–0.6 diopter) in "with-the-rule" astigmatism by all devices and underestimated (0.2–0.3 diopter) in "against-the rule" astigmatism.
Tonn et al[5] (2014)	Pentacam (Oculus, Wetzlar, Germany)	3,818 eyes (2,233 patients)	• Corneal astigmatism from simulated keratometry overestimated total corneal astigmatism in eyes with "with-the-rule" astigmatism. • Total corneal astigmatism could not be predicted by corneal astigmatism from simulated keratometry in eyes that did not have "with-the-rule" astigmatism. • In eyes "with-the-rule" anterior astigmatism, the posterior astigmatism was vertical too in 97%. • In eyes with "against-the-rule" anterior astigmatism, 18% of the cases presented a horizontally oriented posterior astigmatism.

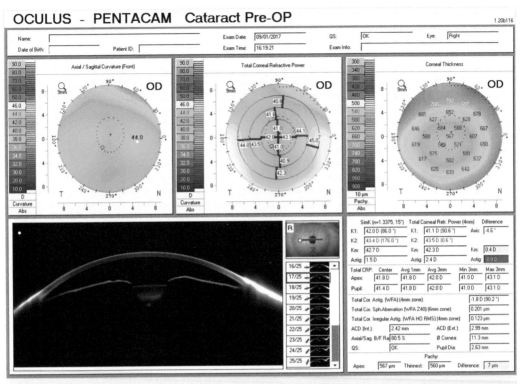

Fig. 5.2 "Cataract preoperative display" available in the Pentacam device. This display allows the surgeon to see the difference between the simulated keratometry (Sim K's) and the total corneal power data, along with thickness metrics and other relevant data derived from corneal and anterior segment tomography.

option is to input the anterior and posterior curvatures in ray tracing thick-lens models like Okulix and PhacoOptics.

The other approach is to use an algorithm that estimates the influence of the posterior astigmatism such as the Baylor nomogram or the Barrett toric calculator. This calculator combines the Universal II Barrett formula to address the effective lens position with a mathematical vector model for PCA (without measuring it), to provide the power and the axis of the toric IOL that should be implanted.

For example, in the case illustrated in ▶ Fig. 5.2, there is ATR astigmatism with front Sim K of + 1.5 diopters of cylinder (CD) at 176 degrees. If Baylor nomogram and AcrySof toric IOL were considered, these data would lead to the implantation of a T5; however, the total corneal power ray-tracing display was + 2.4 CD at 1 degree, which would lead to the implantation of a T6 lens.

Abulafia and coworkers evaluated different methods (Alcon toric calculator, Alcon toric calculator with Baylor nomogram, Holladay toric calculator, Holladay toric calculator with Baylor nomogram, and Barrett Toric IOL Calculator) of measuring and prediction of postoperative astigmatism after toric IOL implantation. Postoperative corneal astigmatism was measured with three different devices (IOLMaster 500, Lenstar LS900, and Atlas topographer). The predicted residual astigmatism at the corneal plane was calculated by the sum of the assumed toric IOL cylinder power at the corneal plane and the measured corneal astigmatism taken by each device. Using vectorial analysis, the error in predicted residual astigmatism was calculated by subtracting the predicted residual astigmatism at the corneal plane from the postoperative subjective refraction at the corneal plane. Absolute and centroid errors were significantly lower with the incorporation of Baylor monogram; from those five methods, Barrett toric calculator provided the lowest results, for both absolute (0.35–0.54 diopters; $p < 0.021$) and centroid (0.01–0.16 diopters; $p < 0.01$) errors. The authors mentioned that the combination of Barrett toric calculator and Lenstar LS 900 achieved the most accurate results (75.0% < 0.50 diopters;

97.1% < 0.75 diopters residual astigmatism).[6] In addition, Reitblat and coworkers and Abulafia and coworkers compared the accuracy of five different strategies to consider posterior corneal curvature in toric IOL calculations: (1) ACA measurements (Lenstar 900); (2) application of Baylor nomogram to ACA measurements; (3) posterior tomography (Pentacam) combined with anterior corneal measurements, using vector summation (vector analysis) as described by Holladay et al; (4) Pentacam true net power calculated using the radii of the anterior and posterior corneal curvatures; and (5) total corneal refractive power calculated using ray tracing by Pentacam.[7] Holladay 2 Consultant Program was chosen to calculate toric IOL power to implant. The median simulated residual astigmatism was lower when vector summation of anterior and posterior astigmatisms (0.49 diopters; $p < 0.001$) was used. Thus, the authors concluded that the combination of PCA (Pentacam) and anterior keratometric measurement (Lenstar 900) might provide lower absolute residual astigmatism results.[8]

Ultimately, Ferreira and coworkers published a study comparing prediction errors in residual astigmatism with all known available methods. IOL spherical power was calculated using the Hoffer Q and SRK/T, according to axial length, < 22.0 and ≥ 22.0 mm, respectively. Lenstar 900, to evaluate corneal astigmatism and curvature, and Pentacam HR, to confirm the regularity of the astigmatism and to evaluate posterior cornea surface, were performed before and after surgery.[9] The IOL cylindrical power was calculated using the manufacturer's (Acrysof IQ Toric SN6AT3-T9, Alcon Laboratories, Inc.) online calculator and Lenstar 900 automated keratometry. They were compared with the methods that take into account predicted effective lens position (ELP; Holladay toric calculator), the methods that consider both ELP and a mathematical model for posterior corneal surface (Barrett toric calculator, Alcon new calculator), the nomograms that consider posterior corneal surface when it is not directly measured (Baylor nomogram, Abulafia–Koch formula, Goggin's coefficient of adjustment), and the Ray-tracing calculation (real posterior corneal surface measurements, PhacoOptics). The Barrett calculator and the newly introduced Alcon calculator yielded the lowest mean absolute and centroid prediction errors (0.30±0.27 and 0.33±0.25 diopters; 0.17 and 0.19 diopters at 165 and 164 degrees, respectively); and on nomogram methods, application of the Abulafia–Koch formula achieved the best results.

The authors concluded that one of these three methods might improve outcomes of toric IOL implantation. In this study, the ray-tracing software failed to obtain a significant lower mean absolute and centroid error (0.57±0.35 and 0.32 diopters at 171, respectively).[9] This illustrates the unquestionable need to evolve in both measurement calculations and modeling optical elements for planning astigmatism treatments with toric IOLs.

5.5 Conclusion

The advent of toric IOLs has significantly improved the optical results of modern cataract surgery. Sim K astigmatism has proved to be relatively inaccurate as target of toric calculations. The main reason is the influence of the PCA whose role and implications have been highlighted by new tomography technologies. It leads to overestimation of the TCA in eyes with WTR astigmatism and underestimation of the TCA in eyes with ATR astigmatism. Nomograms, formulas, and other mathematical models have been developed to overcome this inaccuracy. At the present moment, nomograms and algorithms seem to beat theoretical thick-lens models based on measurements. We anticipate accelerated and significant improvements in every field related to IOL calculations and selections that goes beyond the corneal shape and optics into biomechanical measurements and ocular wavefront aberrometry. These advances will continuously improve the capabilities for minimizing refractive error after cataract surgery, thereby allowing surgeons to improve patient care and patient satisfaction.

5.6 Key Pearls

- The combination of PCA (Pentacam) and anterior keratometric measurement (Lenstar 900) might provide lower absolute residual astigmatism results.
- Due to the influence of the PCA, Sim K astigmatism has proved to be relatively inaccurate as target of toric calculations.
- Failure to include the PCA into calculations leads to incorrect estimation of TCA and unpredictable outcomes.

References

[1] Ambrósio R, Jr, Belin MW. Imaging of the cornea: topography vs tomography. J Refract Surg. 2010; 26(11):847–849
[2] Koch DD, Ali SF, Weikert MP, Shirayama M, Jenkins R, Wang L. Contribution of posterior corneal astigmatism to total

corneal astigmatism. J Cataract Refract Surg. 2012; 38(12): 2080–2087

[3] Savini G, Versaci F, Vestri G, Ducoli P, Næser K. Influence of posterior corneal astigmatism on total corneal astigmatism in eyes with moderate to high astigmatism. J Cataract Refract Surg. 2014; 40(10):1645–1653

[4] Koch DD, Jenkins RB, Weikert MP, Yeu E, Wang L. Correcting astigmatism with toric intraocular lenses: effect of posterior corneal astigmatism. J Cataract Refract Surg. 2013; 39(12): 1803–1809

[5] Tonn B, Klaproth OK, Kohnen T. Anterior surface-based keratometry compared with Scheimpflug tomography-based total corneal astigmatism. Invest Ophthalmol Vis Sci. 2014; 56(1):291–298

[6] Abulafia A, Barrett GD, Kleinmann G, et al. Prediction of refractive outcomes with toric intraocular lens implantation. J Cataract Refract Surg. 2015; 41(5):936–944

[7] Holladay JT, Moran JR, Kezirian GM. Analysis of aggregate surgically induced refractive change, prediction error, and intraocular astigmatism. J Cataract Refract Surg. 2001; 27:61–79

[8] Reitblat O, Levy A, Kleinmann G, Abulafia A, Assia EI. Effect of posterior corneal astigmatism on power calculation and alignment of toric intraocular lenses: comparison of methodologies. J Cataract Refract Surg. 2016; 42(2):217–225

[9] Ferreira TB, Ribeiro P, Ribeiro FJ, O'Neill JG. Comparison of astigmatic prediction errors associated with new calculation methods for toric intraocular lenses. J Cataract Refract Surg. 2017; 43(3):340–347

6 Considerations in Cataract Surgery Following Postrefractive Error Correction

William B. Trattler

Abstract

Considerations in Cataract Surgery Following Postrefractive Error Correction is a chapter that provides surgeons with a comprehensive guide to evaluating and planning cataract surgery in patients who have a history of corneal refractive surgery. Surprisingly, patients with a history of corneal refractive surgery such as LASIK, PRK, or SMILE can have significant differences in their visual results as well as their quality of vision following cataract surgery. This can be related to findings in their preoperative topography, which is detailed in the chapter. Also, a small percentage of post-refractive patients may have ectasia, which is a progressive condition that may require crosslinking before or after cataract surgery. This condition can be identified preoperatively with corneal tomography or topography. With careful preoperative planning, the visual outcomes can be excellent in patients with a history of corneal refractive surgery. However, patients with irregular astigmatism or microstriae should be informed preoperatively that their quality of vision following cataract surgery may be impacted by their pre-existing condition.

Keywords: LASIK, PRK, post-LASIK ectasia, Barrett formula, irregular astigmatism, preoperative topography, preoperative tomography, microstriae, cataract surgery

6.1 Introduction

This chapter deals with all the considerations and precautions that a surgeon should consider in patients who have previously undergone refractive error correction.

There have been significant advances in the preoperative evaluation of the eye prior to cataract surgery, and a number of these advances can help deliver improved outcomes for patients with a history of previous laser corneal refractive surgery, also described as laser vision correction (LVC). This chapter will focus on the evaluation and management of patients with a history of LVC, either laser in situ keratomileusis (LASIK) or photorefractive keratectomy (PRK), as both have a similar impact on the corneal shape. Improvements in intraocular lens (IOL) calculation formulas for patients with a history of LVC have resulted in improvements in visual outcomes following cataract surgery. While most patients can benefit from these technologies and advanced IOL formulas, preoperative imaging technologies can also identify patients who have undergone LVC and have developed irregularities in their corneal shape that can lead to reduced quality of vision following cataract surgery. In comparison to what was available in the past, surgeons have the ability to provide improved visual outcomes to patients with a history of LVC, and also provide education to patients with corneal irregularities as to how their condition may impact their visual results following cataract surgery.

One of the main impacts of LVC on IOL outcomes is related to how LASIK changes the anterior corneal shape of the eye but does not impact the posterior corneal shape. IOL formulas extrapolate the posterior corneal shape based on the power of the anterior cornea. After myopic LVC, the anterior cornea is flatter, and after hyperopic LVC, the anterior cornea is steeper. Using the actual anterior corneal keratometry after LVC in standard IOL formulas results in an incorrect keratometry value, and therefore leads to an incorrect IOL power recommendation. One early method to compensate for this issue was developed by Jack Holladay, MD, and is called the historical method.[1] The historical method requires the pre-LVC keratometry power along with the change in refractive error (as measured at the corneal plane) from before to after LVC. The dioptric power of the refractive change is subtracted from the patient's original keratometry value, which results in an adjusted keratometry value that can be used in standard IOL formulas. One challenge is that over many years and decades, the corneal curvature may differ from the shape of the cornea immediately after LVC, making the historical method less accurate. Also, in many cases, records that provide the original corneal power and change in refraction following LVC are no longer available. Fortunately, more advanced IOL formulas have become available that do not require historical information.

Many studies have looked at the visual outcomes in post-LVC eyes using the many available

IOL formulas. Currently, the Haigis L and the Barrett true K formula appear to provide the best outcomes.[2] However, other formulas can also be used. While the newer formulas provide better outcomes than in the past, there can still be significant variability in postoperative visual results. Therefore, it is important to educate patients with a history of LVC that they are at a higher risk of ending up off target as compared to patients who have not undergone corneal refractive surgery.

6.2 Importance of Preoperative Topography

One of the most important first steps when evaluating a patient with a history of LVC is to perform a topography and/or tomography. Evaluation of these tests is a critical step in determining whether a patient has undergone previous myopic or hyperopic LVC, as well as whether the corneal shape is regular, irregular, or ectatic. ▶ Fig. 6.1 demonstrates the topography of an eye that has previously undergone myopic LASIK. The topography demonstrates a round central flat optical zone surrounded 360 degrees by a red band of elevation. This is a classic appearance of an eye that has undergone previous myopic LVC (either LASIK or PRK). Note that the central Ks are flat. ▶ Fig. 6.2 demonstrates the topography of an eye that has

undergone previous hyperopic LVC. The central cornea is steep. Patients who have undergone hyperopic LVC for very high levels of hyperopia can have an appearance similar to keratoconus (▶ Fig. 6.3). A number of IOL formulas for eyes that have previously undergone LVC, including the Haigis L and Barrett true K, have a specific formula for either hyperopic or myopic LVC, so it is critical to correctly identify which LVC procedure (myopic or hyperopic LVC) a patient has undergone so that the correct IOL formula can be used.

Preoperative topography is also critical, as some patients with a history of previous LVC can develop irregular astigmatism that can impact the quality of vision postoperatively. Identifying this issue preoperatively and discussing with the patient prior to cataract surgery can help set expectations. ▶ Fig. 6.4 shows a topography of an eye that underwent LASIK more than 15 years ago, and now has developed irregular astigmatism that impacts the visual axis. Postoperatively, the patient was very disappointed with her vision and felt that her vision was not improved with cataract surgery. ▶ Fig. 6.5 shows the topography of a patient who previously underwent myopic LASIK, but now has significant irregularity within the visual axis. This patient ended up with reduced UCVA (uncorrected visual acuity) and BCVA (best-corrected visual acuity). It is also important to identify patients who have developed ectasia following LVC.

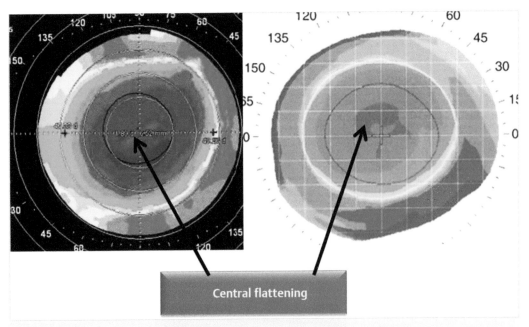

Fig. 6.1 Postmyopic laser in situ keratomileusis. Note the symmetrical area of central flattening.

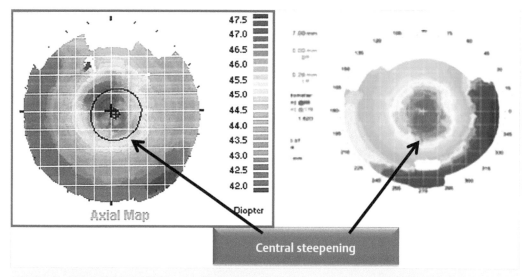

Fig. 6.2 Posthyperopic laser in situ keratomileusis.

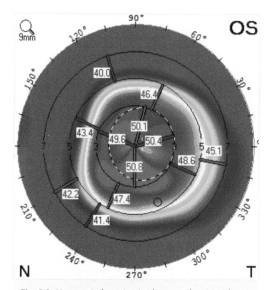

Fig. 6.3 Hyperopic laser in situ keratomileusis with keratoconus pattern.

► Fig. 6.6 demonstrates an eye that had previously undergone LASIK and now has developed post-LASIK ectasia. When ectasia is identified, the cataract surgeon can discuss the treatment options with the patient, which can include cataract surgery first with the future possibility of crosslinking, or crosslinking first followed by cataract surgery either many months or many years later (depending on the cataract severity). One challenge in eyes with ectasia after LASIK is that the traditional post-LASIK IOL calculation formulas are not accurate, and IOL planning reverts toward methods that are used with keratoconus.

One additional challenge in post-LASIK patients is that some patients can have striae or microstriae in the visual axis, which can impact the quality of vision postoperatively. The method for flap creation is a predictor for whether or not microstriae may be present, as metal microkeratome flaps appear to be more commonly associated with microstriae as compared to femtolaser-created flaps. The risk for microstriae in the cornea is also increased in eyes with deeper ablations. For example, in ► Fig. 6.7, the slit-lamp examination reveals microstriae. Even in eyes with a symmetrical topography following myopic LASIK, microstriae can be present, and quality of vision can be affected. While presbyopic IOLs can be used in patients with a history of myopic LASIK, it has been the author's experience that there is an increased chance that a patient can end up less satisfied by their visual result when microstriae are present as compared to similar patients with a history of LASIK that do not have evidence of microstriae in the visual axis.

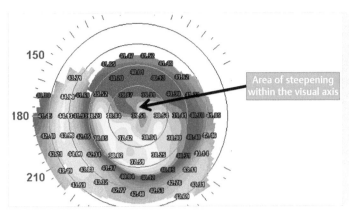

Fig. 6.4 Irregular astigmatism many years after myopic laser in situ keratomileusis.

Area of steepening within the visual axis

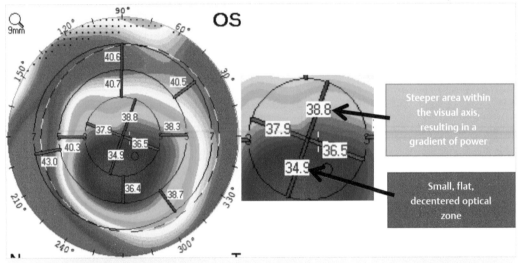

Steeper area within the visual axis, resulting in a gradient of power

Small, flat, decentered optical zone

Fig. 6.5 Irregular astigmatism in the visual axis in a patient with a history of myopic laser in situ keratomileusis for myopia: 38.8 diopters superiorly and 34.9 diopters interiorly.

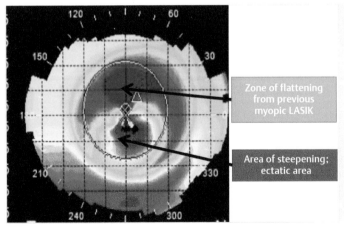

Fig. 6.6 Post laser in situ keratomileusis ectasia in a patient with a visually significant cataract.

Zone of flattening from previous myopic LASIK

Area of steepening; ectatic area

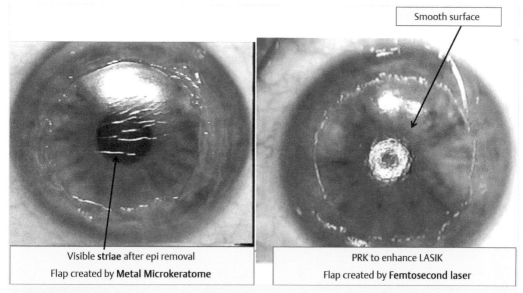

| Visible **striae** after epi removal | PRK to enhance LASIK |
| Flap created by **Metal Microkeratome** | Flap created by **Femtosecond laser** |

Fig. 6.7 Microstriae in the laser in situ keratomileusis flap of a previously myopic patient with a history of a microkeratome flap.

6.3 Optimizing Visual Outcomes in Post-LASIK Patients

Determining the optimal IOL power in patients who have previously undergone LASIK is a challenge, even with modern formulas. One important step in the preoperative planning is to obtain reliable keratometry for the IOL calculation formulas. A high percentage of patients scheduled for cataract surgery have dry eye, so dry eye/ocular surface disease needs to be identified and treated prior to obtaining final biometry readings.[3] Once optimal biometry readings have been captured, the data can be imported into a latest-generation IOL formula for the post-LASIK patient. Many of the formulas are available at no cost for use on ophthalmology organization websites. For example, the ASCRS (American Society of Cataract and Refractive Surgery) website provides one data entry form, and runs numerous post-LASIK IOL calculation formulas. One challenge is that transferring data from a biometry device to an online calculator increases the risk of a transcription error. Many biometry devices have integrated post-Lasik IOL formulas, which helps avoid the risk of a transcription error. The Barrett true K and Haigis-L appear to provide the best outcomes.[4] Some surgeons employ interoperative wavefront

aberrometry to help optimize the IOL power.[4] However, even with these tools and technologies, a small percentage of patients will end up significantly off target, so educating patients on this potential risk can help manage expectations. If a patient ends up off target, they can consider various surgical options for improving their uncorrected vision, including an IOL exchange, piggyback IOL, or PRK with mitomycin C over the previous LASIK flap. They can of course consider nonsurgical options including spectacles or contact lenses.

6.4 Conclusion

In summary, significant progress has been made in providing excellent visual outcomes to patients with a history of LVC who require cataract surgery. Using the latest postrefractive surgery, IOL formulas can help minimize the risk that a patient ends up significantly off target. It is of course important to carefully evaluate the preoperative topography or tomography to identify whether the patient had previous myopic or hyperopic LASIK, as well as to determine whether the cornea has a regular shape, or has evidence of irregularity, especially within the visual axis. If ectasia is discovered, management of this condition should be discussed with the patient. Importantly, ocular surface disease should be identified and managed to help optimize the biometry readings in advance of surgery. With these points in mind, surgeons can help improve their patients' chances of ending up with a good visual outcome following cataract surgery.

6.5 Key Pearls

- A preoperative topography and/or tomography can determine whether a patient has undergone previous myopic or hyperopic laser vision correction, as well as determine whether the corneal shape is regular, irregular, or ectatic.
- While newer formulas provide better visual outcomes than in the past, there can still be significant variability in postoperative visual results in patients with a history of laser vision correction.
- Topography can reveal patients who have developed irregular astigmatism, which will negatively impact quality of vision following cataract surgery.

- If preoperative topography identifies post-LASIK ectasia, surgeons can consider whether to perform cataract surgery first, or corneal crosslinking prior to cataract surgery.
- IOL formulas developed for patients with a history of laser vision correction may not provide accurate IOL recommendations in patients with post-LASIK ectasia.

References

[1] Holladay JT. Consultations in refractive surgery. Refract Corneal Surg. 1989; 5:203

[2] Hamed AM, Wang L, Misra M, Koch DD. A comparative analysis of five methods of determining corneal refractive power in eyes that have undergone myopic laser in situ keratomileusis. Ophthalmology. 2002; 109(4):651–658

[3] Ianchulev T, Hoffer KJ, Yoo SH, et al. Intraoperative refractive biometry for predicting intraocular lens power calculation after prior myopic refractive surgery. Ophthalmology. 2014; 121(1):56–60

[4] Fram NR, Masket S, Wang L. Comparison of intraoperative aberrometry, OCT-based IOL formula, Haigis-L, and Masket formulae for IOL power calculation after laser vision correction. Ophthalmology. 2015; 122(6):1096–1101

Part II

Refractive Enhancement Procedures

7 Corneal-Based Procedures: Astigmatic Keratotomy, LASIK, PRK, and SMILE

Jennifer Loh and William B. Trattler

Abstract

Corneal-Based Procedures: Astigmatic Keratotomy, LASIK, PRK, and SMILE is a chapter that is focused on the correction of residual refractive error in patients who have previously undergone cataract surgery. While improvements in IOL calculations have resulted in a higher percentage of patients with excellent uncorrected vision after cataract surgery, there are still a small percentage of patients who have residual refractive error that results in unsatisfactory uncorrected vision. Patients can consider a variety of options to improve their vision, including glasses, contact lenses, intraocular surgery, and corneal refractive surgery. This chapter focuses on the preoperative evaluation and corneal refractive surgery options for patients who desire improvement in their uncorrected vision. While all surgeries carry a small degree of risk, the overall risks with corneal refractive surgery is on the low side, making this an appropriate option for patients who desire improvement in their vision and understand that there are uncommon but serious risks with surgery. The chapter should help the cataract and refractive surgeon in the evaluation and management of patients, and hopefully lead to successful visual outcomes.

Keywords: LASIK, PRK, SMILE, enhancement, EBK, cataract surgery, pseudophakia

7.1 Introduction

This chapter deals with the technique of corneal-based refractive procedures for the correction of residual refractive error. It will also highlight the application of femtosecond lasers for achieving precision and predictable results by customizing the incisions for reproducible results. The shortcomings of the procedure will also be highlighted, as all the patients who need an enhancement procedure are not suited for a corneal touch-up procedure.

7.2 Exceeding Patient Expectations for Cataract Surgery

Expectations for exceptional vision after cataract surgery are very high, especially in patients who have healthy eyes prior to surgery. Over the last two decades, cataract surgery has become both a vision restoration procedure and a vision optimization procedure. Patients who have worn glasses and contact lenses their entire lives can experience a reduced need for vision correction following cataract surgery. However, despite wonderful outcomes for the vast majority of patients, there is a small percentage of patients who end up dissatisfied with their visual results, as they require spectacles or contact lenses to achieve satisfactory vision. When the cause of the dissatisfaction is due to residual refractive error after cataract surgery, it is fortunate that there are a number of surgical and nonsurgical options to improve vision. It is of course important to evaluate patients and determine whether patients are appropriate candidates for vision correction procedures.

The ability for cataract surgeons to leave patients with minimal refractive error has improved over the past decade. First, evidence was developed that a high percentage of patients presenting for cataract surgery had preexisting dry eye, resulting in reduced accuracy of preoperative corneal shape measurements.[1] When preoperative tests reveal telltale signs of inaccuracy, patients can be treated for dry eye, and return for repeat measurements 2 to 4 weeks later (▶ Fig. 7.1, ▶ Fig. 7.2). A second improvement for surgeons has been advancements in intraocular lens (IOL) calculation formulas. The latest-generation formulas, including the Hill-radial basis function and Barrett Universal II provide improved visual outcomes over a wide range of axial lengths, corneal steepness values, and anterior chamber depth.[2] A third improvement over the past decade has been intraoperative aberrometry, which surgeons

Pre-op topography

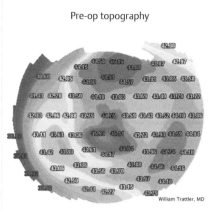

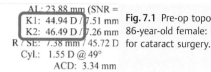

AL: 23.88 mm (SNR =
K1: 44.94 D / 7.51 mm
K2: 46.49 D / 7.26 mm
R / SE: 7.38 mm / 45.72 D
Cyl.: 1.55 D @ 49°
ACD: 3.34 mm

Status: Phakic

Fig. 7.1 Pre-op topography of an 86-year-old female: initial consultation for cataract surgery.

TECNIS MF1 ONE
ZMB00

A const:	119.3
IOL (D)	REF (D)
20.5	-1.55
20.0	-1.23
19.5	-0.91
19.0	-0.59
18.5	-0.28
18.0	0.03
17.5	0.34

William Trattler, MD

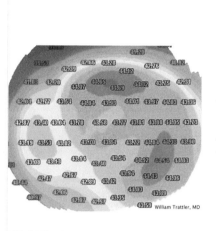

AL: 23.93 mm (SNR =
K1: 43.55 D / 7.75 mm
K2: 43.89 D / 7.69 mm
R / SE: 7.72 mm / 43.72 D
Cyl.: 0.34 D @ 103°
ACD: 3.25 mm

Status: Phakic

Fig. 7.2 Dry eye identified 1 month later after topical steroids for 1 week and cyclosporine twice daily for 1 month. Two-diopter shift in intraocular lens power (from 18.5 to 20.5 diopters).

TECNIS MF1 ONE
ZMB00

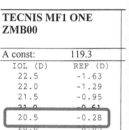

A const:	119.3
IOL (D)	REF (D)
22.5	-1.63
22.0	-1.29
21.5	-0.95
21.0	-0.61
20.5	-0.28
20.0	0.05
19.5	0.38

William Trattler, MD

report can significantly improve visual outcomes.[3] All of these advances have helped improve the chance a patient will end up on target, but there are still a small percentage of patients who remain off target and unhappy with their visual outcomes.

7.3 Preoperative Evaluation of Pseudophakic Patients

Evaluation of pseudophakic patients who desire improvement in their refractive outcomes starts with a measurement of their uncorrected vision, best-corrected vision, and refractive error. Slit-lamp examination with a careful evaluation for ocular surface disease including dry eye, corneal

staining, and blepharitis is critical in helping determine whether the patient is ready to consider a refractive enhancement, or whether therapy for underlying conditions is required. If epithelial membrane dystrophy is present and thought to be impacting visual results, an epithelial debridement procedure can be considered to normalize the corneal shape before embarking on a definitive treatment for the residual refractive error (▶ Fig. 7.3). Corneal thickness should be measured, as well as intraocular pressure (IOP). A dilated examination is also important to identify posterior capsular opacity, as well as the IOL location and centration. Optical coherence tomography (OCT) of the macula can be performed to identify patients with macular conditions such as epiretinal membranes,

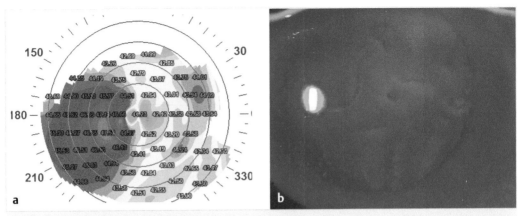

Fig. 7.3 Epithelial basement membrane dystrophy causing irregular astigmatism and reduced best-corrected visual acuity (BCVA). **(a)** Irregular astigmatism on topography with pseudophakia, BCVA = 20/30, and normal macular optical coherence tomography (OCT). **(b)** Epithelial basement membrane dystrophy (EBMD).

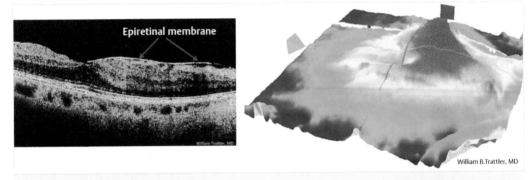

Fig. 7.4 Optical coherence tomography as a test prior to cataract surgery may reveal an epiretinal membrane (ERM).

vitreomacular traction, or other issues that can also be impacting a patient's satisfaction with their vision (▶ Fig. 7.4).

Corneal topography and/or tomography are critical tests for patients with residual refractive errors who are being considered for corneal refractive surgery. Of note, even if a corneal map was performed prior to cataract surgery, it is important to perform a map during the postoperative period prior to performing corneal refractive surgery, as the map may have changed following surgery. The corneal mapping will help determine whether patients are candidates for corneal refractive surgery, including laser in situ keratomileusis (LASIK), small incision lenticule extraction (SMILE), photo-refractive keratectomy (PRK), and/or astigmatic keratotomy (AK).

Following the testing, patients can be informed of their options. While it may seem obvious, patients should be informed that options for improving their vision include nonsurgical options such as contact lenses and glasses. If patients express a desire for a surgical option to improve their vision, patients can receive information on procedures that include IOL exchange, piggyback IOL, as well as various corneal refractive procedures. Patients are often candidates for more than one procedure, and a discussion of the risks, benefits, and visual expectations can help both the surgeon and patient decide on the best course of action. For example, if a patient has previously had a yttrium aluminum garnet (YAG) capsulotomy, a piggyback IOL, or corneal refractive procedure may be lower risk as compared to an IOL exchange with an open capsule. On the other hand, if a patient has 3 diopters of hyperopia and has an intact capsule, performing an IOL exchange or piggyback IOL can be quite effective and may provide superior visual results than LASIK, PRK, or SMILE. It is important to point out that some patients may not be appropriate candidates for corneal refractive procedures, such as patients with keratoconus, pellucid marginal degeneration, or post-LASIK ectasia, and therefore IOL exchange or piggyback IOL may be a patient's only option if they are dissatisfied with their visual result.

In most cases, corneal refractive surgery can be an appropriate and effective option for enhancing a patient's vision following cataract surgery. Generally, there is only a small residual refractive error in pseudophakic patients who desire better uncorrected vision, which means that the amount of treatment to the cornea required is on the lower side in these cases compared to the typical patient undergoing corneal refractive surgery. However, one major challenge is that pseudophakic patients tend to be significantly older than patients who have not undergone cataract surgery. In a retrospective study looking at outcomes of PRK in patients with residual refractive error following cataract surgery, the average age of my patients was 65 years.[4] Patients who are in their 60 s and 70 s are more likely to have dry eye, which can impact the speed of epithelial healing. However, once dry eye has been addressed, pseudophakic patients can expect very good outcomes with corneal refractive surgery.

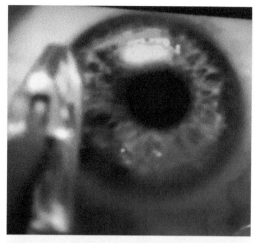

Fig. 7.5 Epithelial Bowman's keratomileusis surface ablation procedure.

7.4 Corneal Refractive Procedure Options

Once patients have decided to move forward with treatment, the surgeon can evaluate the patient and determine which corneal refractive procedure (if any) would work best for a particular patient. One of the main decision points revolves around the refractive error. If the patient has myopia with low astigmatism, PRK, LASIK, and SMILE are excellent choices for the patient and the surgeon. While LASIK and SMILE have the advantage of providing very rapid visual recovery, their downside is that some cataract surgeons may not be as experienced with these procedures. On the other hand, innovations with the PRK procedure can help lead to a more rapid visual recovery compared to previous techniques. For example, epithelial Bowman's keratomileusis (EBK) uses a new soft plastic spatula for epithelial removal that has been found to result in better vision during the first few days after surgery, and a more rapid visual recovery (▶ Fig. 7.5). PRK may be the corneal refractive procedure of

choice for patients with previous PRK, LASIK, SMILE, or radial keratotomy (RK), as the PRK procedure may be less invasive than LASIK or SMILE for these patients. Overall, PRK, LASIK, and SMILE can be expected to effectively reduce the refractive error in pseudophakic patients, resulting in improved vision postoperatively.

Some pseudophakic patients may have a low refractive error with mild to moderate astigmatism, and spherical equivalent close to the target refraction. In these cases, corneal relaxing procedures such as AK or limbal relaxing incisions (LRIs) may be the procedure of choice. When assessing patients for candidacy for corneal relaxing procedures, it is important to evaluate the topography and exclude patients who may have corneal ectatic conditions such as keratoconus or pellucid. The AK procedure can be performed manually with a blade, or with a femtosecond laser. The advantage of corneal relaxing procedures is that they provide very rapid visual recovery and are very low risk. With a nomogram, these procedures typically provide improved vision. However, one downside is that in the short term patients can end up undercorrected, while in the long term (many years), some patients can have continued refractive effect of the incisions, leading to overcorrection.

7.5 Conclusion

In summary, corneal refractive procedures are an effective option for patients who have undergone lens replacement surgery but have residual refractive error. Identifying appropriate candidates is critical, as this will result in better postoperative outcomes. Also, alternative procedures, including IOL exchange and piggyback IOLs, may be better options for patients with certain postoperative refractions, as well as patients who have preoperative conditions such as keratoconus or patients who have already previously undergone significant corneal refractive surgery. For patients who are appropriate candidates, PRK, LASIK, SMILE, and AK can all be effective tools for providing improved uncorrected vision, and therefore can be considered for patients who are dissatisfied by their visual outcomes following both cataract surgery and elective lens replacement surgeries.

7.6 Key Pearls

- Patients dissatisfied with their vision following cataract surgery can undergo evaluation to determine whether they are eligible for corneal refractive surgery to improve their vision.
- Identify and treat corneal conditions such as ocular surface disease and EBMD prior to performing corneal refractive surgery, as the vision and refractive error may improve with treatment.

- LASIK, SMILE and PRK are all effective corneal refractive surgeries for enhancing the vision in pseudophakic patients.
- Epithelial Bowman's keratomileusis (EBK) uses a new soft plastic spatula for epithelial removal that results in better vision during the first few days after surgery, and a more rapid visual recovery as compared to standard PRK.
- While corneal refractive surgery is often the best choice, some patients may be better candidates for intraocular procedures, such as piggyback IOLs and IOL exchanges.

References

[1] Trattler WB, Majmudar PA, Donnenfeld ED, McDonald MB, Stonecipher KG, Goldberg DF. The Prospective Health Assessment of Cataract Patients' Ocular Surface (PHACO) study: the effect of dry eye. Clin Ophthalmol. 2017; 11:1423–1430
[2] Melles RB, Holladay JT, Chang WJ. Accuracy of intraocular lens calculation formulas. Ophthalmology. 2018; 125(2): 169–178
[3] Hatch KM, Woodcock EC, Talamo JH. Intraocular lens power selection and positioning with and without intraoperative aberrometry. J Refract Surg. 2015; 31(4):237–242
[4] Khell J, Kaiser C, Spektor F, Liss E, Trattler W, Buznego C. Comparative Evaluation of PRK and LASiK for Vision Enhancement After Implantation of Presbyopic IOL; Poster presented at ARVO Annual Meeting; March 2012

8 Intraocular Lens Exchange

Thomas A. Oetting

Abstract

This chapter deals with the method, technique, and difficulties encountered in intraocular lens (IOL) exchange when adopted for residual refractive error correction and for other reasons. It is often necessary to exchange an IOL and the reasons can vary from placement of wrong power of IOL to decentrations and dislocations. Depending on the clinical scenario, the surgeon should be well versed with the various techniques of IOL exchange. This chapter highlights the causes and the surgical details that the surgeon should be acquainted with in order to perform a successful IOL exchange.

Keywords: IOL exchange, IOL scaffold, decentered IOL, IOL cutting, IOL explantation, IOL insertion

8.1 Introduction

Occasionally an intraocular lens (IOL) must be exchanged as the IOL may have simply been the wrong power or is not tolerated due to glare or dysphotopsia. The IOL may have opacified with time; or most commonly, the IOL may have become unstable or subluxed due to progressive zonular laxity[1] or the IOL may be causing inflammation, uveitis, hemorrhage, or ocular hypertension.[2] Removing an IOL can be difficult due to the development of adhesions, especially if it has been in place for several years.[3] This chapter outlines the indications for IOL exchange with an emphasis on explantation and capsular placement, as other chapters discuss the techniques for IOL implantation without capsular support.

8.2 Indications for Intraocular Lens Exchange

Dr. Nick Mamalis and his colleagues at the University of Utah produced a classic paper on the indications for explanted IOLs. In this paper, the indications for IOL explantation depend on the type of IOL (▶ Table 8.1) with IOL explantation most common in dislocated or decentered single-piece acrylic (SPA) IOL.[1] The strategy for and the issues surrounding explantation differ depending on the reason for explantation.

8.2.1 Refractive

In many ways, the simplest indication for IOL exchange comes when the wrong power of IOL is placed inside the eye. It may be difficult to explain to the patient why the surgical team placed the wrong power IOL, but the actual surgery is relatively easy. The surgery is straightforward as the error is often detected early in the postoperative course. As such, the haptics are not yet excessively adherent to the capsule that allows one to easily free the IOL from the capsule. Freeing the IOL, especially the IOL haptics, is the most difficult part of an IOL exchange.

Jin et al prepared a nice series of cases where the wrong power of IOL was placed. They showed that the most common reason for placing the wrong power of IOL was incorrect estimation of the corneal power, followed by incorrect axial length measurement and thus followed by simply placing the incorrect IOL.[2] The time from original surgery to the exchange varied from 1 day to 14 months with an average of 2.6 months.[2] Following exchange in their series, 95% of patients had a best-corrected visual acuity of better than 20/40.[2] Another option in patients with the wrong power IOL is to use refractive corneal surgery rather than lens exchange.[3]

Table 8.1 Intraocular lens (IOL) explantation by IOL type

IOL type	Primary explantation: indication	Percent of IOLs explanted
Single-piece acrylic	Dislocation/ decentration	24
Multifocal acrylic	Visual aberration	23
Three-piece silicon	Visual aberration	20
Three-piece acrylic	Incorrect IOL power	19
Single-piece silicon	Dislocation/ decentration	6

Source: Adapted from Mamalis N, Brubaker J, Davis D, Espandar L, Werner L. Complications of foldable intraocular lenses requiring explantation or secondary intervention–2007 survey update. J Cataract Refract Surg 2008;34(9):1584–1591.

8.2.2 Visual Aberration

Visual aberrations such as glare disturbances, halos, and dysphotopsia are a common indication for IOL exchange, especially with multifocal IOLs.[1] Unlike the situation where the wrong power IOL is placed, the decision to remove the IOL with visual aberrations is often delayed as the surgeon waits for symptoms to resolve.[4] As a result, removing these lenses can be difficult as the capsule may be more adherent to the optic and more importantly to the haptics. In addition, it can be difficult to determine if the symptoms are related to the IOL, the wound, or the posterior capsule.

Davison reported on a large series of acrylic IOLs and described the positive and negative dysphotopsia with these popular square edge optic high refractive index IOLs.[5] However, these visual aberrations have been associated with most of the IOLs in use including the rounded three-piece silicon IOLs.[1] Geneva and Henderson nicely outlined the difficulty with treating negative dysphotopsia.[6] In general, positive dysphotopsia are more associated with square edge lenses and the high index IOL materials, and the exchange strategy is to replace the existing IOL with one of a different material. In general, negative dysphotopsia is associated with high index IOL material and a square edge, and the strategy is to place the new IOL more anteriorly in the sulcus or with the optic anteriorly captured by the anterior capsule.

8.2.3 Inappropriate Intraocular Lens in the Sulcus

A perfect sulcus IOL would have a large optic (6 mm or greater), long thin haptics (14 mm or greater), and has smooth anterior optic surface to lessen iris irritation. In addition, avoiding silicon may be of some benefit if the patient is at risk for the future placement of silicon oil or an air–fluid exchange during pars plana vitrectomy, as the silicon lenses can cloud with these procedures. Most of the three-piece IOLs in the U.S. market have haptics that are too short (13 mm). We reported on our experience with the Alcon MA50 three-piece acrylic IOL with a 6.5-mm optic, which worked well except in long eyes where the 13.0-mm haptic length was not long enough to ensure centration.[7]

Unfortunately, not all IOLs placed in the sulcus are suited for sulcus placement. The popularity of SPA IOLs has led some to place SPA IOLs in the sulcus either inadvertently or when presented with an intraocular complication such as a posterior capsular tear. Dr. David Chang and the cataract clinical committee of the American Society of Cataract and Refractive Surgery (ASCRS) reported on a series of patients with poorly placed SPA IOLs.[8] In this series, at least one of the SPA haptics was in the sulcus. The thick square edged haptics of the SPA IOLs placed in the sulcus led to a variety of problems including chronic uveitis, glaucoma, and hemorrhage.

The surgical strategy for eliminating the problems associated with SPA IOLs in the sulcus involves removing the thick SPA haptic from the sulcus either by repositioning the IOL such that both haptics are in the capsular bag or by removing the SPA IOL and exchanging for a large three-piece IOL better suited for the sulcus. In several cases in Chang et al's series of misplaced SPA IOLS, one haptic was in the bag and the other was in the sulcus. In this situation, ophthalmic viscoelastic devices (OVD) should be used to separate the haptic from the bag to allow explantation of the SPA.[8] Samuel Masket has described the technique (personal communication) of simply cutting off and removing the sulcus-based haptic and leaving the remaining portions of the SPA in the capsular bag. In some cases, you may be able to reform the capsular bag with OVD and position the sulcus haptic into its proper location in the bag.

8.2.4 Dislocation/Decentration Intraocular Lens

The most common reason for IOL explantation is decentration or dislocation.[1] Decentration is when the IOL is in the proper plane, but not centered. Decentration, especially when it occurs early in the postoperative period, is often caused by inadvertent placement of one haptic in the sulcus and one in the bag. Occasionally, decentration can be caused by a damaged haptic, but this is less common especially with the commonly used SPA IOLs. Decentration of IOLs with both haptics placed in the sulcus is more common when the IOL haptics are too short for sulcus placement (< 12.5 mm). Dislocation of IOLs where the IOL may also be too posterior or loose (pseudophacodonesis) is typically caused by areas of weakened zonules, which can occur even years after implantation.

Rather than explanting a decentered IOL, often the best strategy is to secure or reposition the existing IOL (▶ Table 8.2). Sometimes the IOL can simply be repositioned and secured using the existing remnant of the capsule. More often, the

Table 8.2 Intraocular lens (IOL) decentration

IOL location	Typical cause of decentration	Exchange strategy	Secure existing IOL strategy
Both haptics in secure capsular bag	Capsular phimosis Damaged haptic Both haptics are not really in bag	Free IOL from capsule and remove IOL New IOL in sulcus	Free IOL from capsule and suture to iris Modify anterior capsule
Both haptics in loose capsular bag (dislocation)	Zonular weakness	Remove capsule and IOL through large incision Free IOL from capsule and remove IOL New IOL AC, glued	Suture IOL/capsule to sclera Free IOL from capsule suture to iris Free IOL from capsule Suture/glue to sclera
Three-piece IOL One haptic in bag one in sulcus	Not placed properly	Free optic and one haptic from capsule and remove most of IOL New IOL in sulcus	Free optic and haptic from bag and leave in sulcus
SPA IOL One haptic in bag one in sulcus	Not placed properly	Free optic and one haptic from capsule and remove most of IOL New IOL in sulcus	Separate capsule And place both haptics in bag Cut off offending haptic and leave remainder in bag
Three-piece IOL Both haptics in sulcus	IOL too small Zonular weakness	IOL is usually free New IOL large three piece	Suture IOL to iris Glue IOL to sclera (Agarwal's technique) Suture IOL to sclera
SPA Both haptics in sulcus	Not placed properly	IOL is usually free New IOL three piece in sulcus or traditional optic capture	Separate capsule And place both haptics in bag

Abbreviations: AC, anterior chamber; Glued IOL, glue-assisted intrascleral haptic fixation of an IOL; SPA, single-piece acrylic.
Adapted from Oetting TA. Explanting a posterior chamber intraocular lens. In: Agarwal A, Narang P, eds. Phacoemulsification. New Delhi: JayPee Highlights Medical Publisher; 2012:510–515

decentered IOL is freed from capsular remnants and sutured to the iris or sclera or glued to the sclera as outlined in Chapter 14. If it is possible to secure the existing IOL, this is usually the best approach as it minimizes the trauma to the eye that comes with an exchange of the IOL.

One of the most difficult situations presents when the IOL is in the bag, but the bag itself is loose. This situation seems to be more common as we operate sooner on patients who live longer. This is especially noted in patients with pseudoexfoliation, uveitis, trauma, or other conditions with weakened zonules. The surgeon has three choices in this situation: suture the IOL and the bag to the sclera, remove the IOL from the bag and secure the IOL only to the sclera or iris, or finally explant the IOL. The choice depends on the type of IOL, the amount of residual lens material in the capsular bag with the IOL, and the age of the patient.

8.2.5 Uveitis–Glaucoma–Hyphema Syndrome

The uveitis–glaucoma–hyphema (UGH) syndrome is related to uveal tissue in contact with an IOL. Uveal inflammation in the UGH syndrome seems to come from contact of the IOL (usually the haptics) to the iris or ciliary body. The hyphema or vitreous hemorrhage comes from episodic injury to vessels in the iris, ciliary body, or angle. The glaucoma is secondary to the uveitis, treatment of the uveitis, pigment dispersion, hemorrhage, or direct injury to angle structures.

When anterior chamber (AC) IOLs were commonly placed, the UGH syndrome was the second most common indication for IOL exchange behind bullous keratopathy.[2] As posterior chamber (PC) IOLs began to dominate our practice, the UGH syndrome became less common, but still important.

PC IOLs in the sulcus are at the most risk for UGH syndrome, especially if they are loose[7] or are SPA IOLs with wide square haptics.[8] Even PC IOLs positioned completely in the capsular bag can cause the UGH syndrome if the zonules are loose and the resultant pseudophacodonesis irritates the iris. The author typically will exchange an AC IOL for a posterior IOL causing UGH and similarly will exchange a posterior IOL for an AC IOL causing UGH.

8.3 Freeing the Existing Intraocular Lens from the Capsule

The ease of IOL removal is mostly dependent on how long the IOL has been in the bag. IOLs that have been in the bag for a few weeks, such as when the wrong IOL is placed, are very easy to free from the bag. IOLs that have been in the bag for years, such as with opacified IOLs, can be very hard to remove. Removing an IOL with an intact posterior capsule is far easier than when the patient has had a yttrium aluminum garnet (YAG) posterior capsulotomy. When the IOL is in the sulcus, it is typically not adherent to the capsule and can easily be removed.

The first step to free the IOL from the bag is to somehow get a dissection plane started between

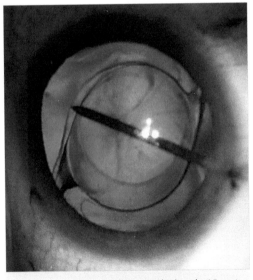

Fig. 8.1 A 27-gauge needle is attached to the Viscoat syringe and the sharp end of the needle is used to get under the capsule and then inject the ophthalmic viscoelastic device to start the viscodissection.

the IOL and the capsule. The author likes to use a viscous and dispersive OVD (e.g., Viscoat) especially when the posterior capsule is not intact. With IOLs that have been in place for a while (e.g., more than a year) it is advisable to use a 27-gauge needle attached to the Viscoat syringe and use the sharp end of the needle to get under the capsule and then inject the OVD to start the dissection (▶ Fig. 8.1). Sometimes the author uses the micro forceps (such as the Microsurgical Technology [MST] Duet micro forceps) to lift the capsule to allow a cannula to get access under the AC that allows vigorous viscodissection (▶ Fig. 8.2). The author also like to use a flat hydrodissection cannula attached to the OVD syringe for viscodissection, as the flat surface of the cannula makes it easier to get between the capsule and the IOL yet still allows for vigorous flow of the OVD.

When freeing the IOL, most of the surgeon's attention should be directed to freeing up the haptics with viscodissection. If the posterior capsule is intact, the OVD will often track around the optic that makes freeing the optic of its posterior attachments fairly easy. However, freeing the haptics can often be very difficult. A generous use of OVD dissection should be adopted to separate the anterior and posterior capsule in the area of the two haptics and carry the viscodissection as posterior as possible. When you think you have freed the capsular adhesions to the haptics, try to spin the IOL clockwise to allow the haptics to work free of the capsule. Sometimes the haptics are just too stuck and must be cut to be free of the IOL. Often the cut haptic can be left in the bag and the remainder of the IOL can be removed. Sometimes the cut haptics will come out more easily without the optic as you may have a better angle to removing the

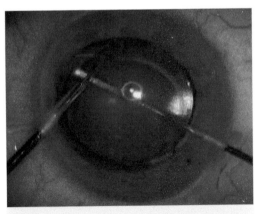

Fig. 8.2 Forceps to help with viscodissection.

haptic through tunnels formed by adhesion of the anterior and posterior capsules.

8.4 Strategies to Remove the Intraocular Lens

8.4.1 Crafting a New 6-mm Incision

Sometimes the most efficient strategy is to simply make a 6.0-mm incision to remove the freed IOL. Polymethyl meth acrylate (PMMA) IOL optics is difficult to cut as the IOL often tilts and the material can splinter, which makes removing them whole as the most elegant strategy. PMMA IOLs would include older PC IOLs, AC IOLs, and eyelet haptic IOLs like the CZ70. PMMA IOL optics are

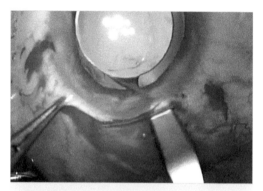

Fig. 8.3 Making a 6-mm scleral tunnel for intraocular lens explantation.

usually 6 to 7 mm and if the surgeon plans to perform an exchange and place an AC IOL, then it is essential to make a large incision for IOL insertion.

A well-crafted short scleral tunnel incision that is approximately 6.0 mm in length is very stable. The author would suggest making a peritomy and applying cautery. Use a crescent blade to produce a one-third scleral depth scleral tunnel that is very close to the limbus centrally and about 1 mm posterior at either end of the 6-mm tunnel (▶ Fig. 8.3). Prepare the incision before entering the eye so the eye is firm while crafting the short tunnel. Two or three interrupted 10–0 nylon sutures will easily close a well-constructed tunnel.

8.4.2 Refolding the Intraocular Lens

The acrylic IOLs with high index of refraction (e.g., MA60, SA60, and SNWF) can be refolded within the eye using folding forceps through the clear corneal wound. The typical refolding technique uses a paracentesis across from the main wound (3.5 mm) to introduce a spatula to place under the optic while using an open IOL insertion forceps above the optic in the AC (▶ Table 8.3). While lifting with the spatula and coming down on top of the optic with the open insertion forceps, the IOL can be folded in the AC (▶ Fig. 8.4). Dispersive viscoelastic is placed above and below the optic to protect the capsule and the corneal endothelium. Once folded, the IOL is simply removed through the 3.5-mm wound. Refolding the IOL only works

Table 8.3 Removing intraocular lens (IOLs)

IOL type	Removal technique	Example
SPA AcrySof	Refold in anterior chamber (AC); remove with 3.5- to 4-mm wound Henderson's technique (3 mm) Cut in AC (3 mm)	SN60WF SA60AT
Three-piece AcrySof	Refold in AC; remove with 3.5- to 4-mm wound Cut in AC (3 mm)	MA60AT
Other foldable (all materials)	Cut in AC (3 mm)	AR40 SI30 CQ2015
Plate haptic (silicon or collamer)	Cut in AC (3 mm) Henderson's technique (3 mm)	Nanoflex
Calcified opaque foldable IOL	Create 6.0-mm wound	
PMMA	Create 6.0-mm wound	AC IOL

Abbreviations: PMMA, poly methyl methacrylate; SPA, single-piece acrylic.
Source: Adapted from Oetting TA. Explanting a posterior chamber intraocular lens. In: Agarwal A, Narang P, eds. Phacoemulsification. New Delhi: JayPee Highlights Medical Publisher; 2012:510–515

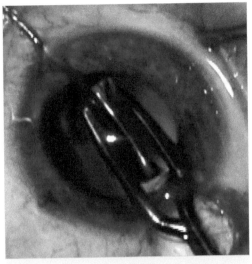

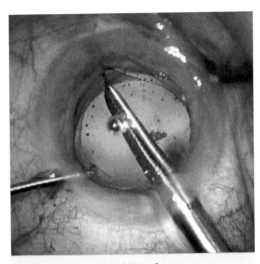

Fig. 8.6 Osher cutter with Duet forceps.

Fig. 8.4 Intraocular lens folding inside the eye.

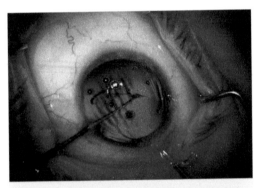

Fig. 8.5 Removal of the intraocular lens according to Dr. Henderson's technique by pulling on an externalized haptic (with 0.12 or similar toothed forceps) through a 2.5- to 3.0-mm wound while pushing on the optic 180 degrees across from the wound (inside the eye) with a hook.

well with thin acrylic IOLs like the single- and three-piece Alcon AcrySof IOLs and in the hands, is virtually impossible with thick acrylic IOLs (e.g., AR40) and slippery IOLs like the silicon three-piece IOLs (e.g., SI30).

An interesting refolding technique comes from Bonnie Henderson (Ophthalmic Consultants of Boston) for folding high index of refraction (i.e., thin) SPA IOLs such as the Alcon SN60WF IQ. Dr.

Henderson's technique is to simply pull on an externalized haptic (with 0.12 or similar toothed forceps) through a 2.5- to 3.0-mm wound while pushing on the optic 180 degrees across from the wound (inside the eye) with a hook (▶ Fig. 8.5). For some reason, amazingly and almost magically, the IOL folds itself and pops out of the eye. Plate haptic silicon IOLs can also be removed in a similar fashion.

8.4.3 Cutting the Intraocular Lens

There are several ways to cut an IOL to get the optic small enough to remove through a small incision. One classic technique is to only cut about two-thirds through the IOL and make what looks like a "Pac Man" and rotate the IOL out through the wound. The more common technique is to simply cut the IOL completely in half or into thirds and bring out the pieces. The author likes the Osher mildly serrated cutter from Duckworth and Kent (▶ Fig. 8.6). You can usually keep the IOL from flopping around too much by holding the externalized haptic with this cutter. The author also really likes to use the MST Duet micro forceps through a paracentesis to hold the IOL while cutting it through the main incision with MST IOL cutters. The forceps help make sure that IOL tilting does not cause corneal damage while cutting the IOL (▶ Fig. 8.7). If you are in a bind, you can even use Vannas scissors to cut most IOLs.

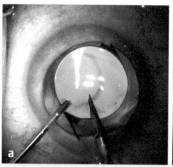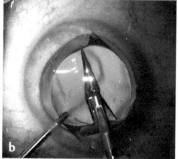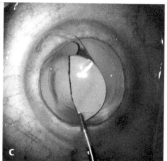

Fig. 8.7 Intraocular lens (IOL) cutting **(a,b)** Duet forceps to cut the IOL in half. **(c)** Duet forceps cut the IOL in half removing the last half.

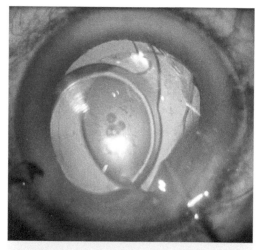

Fig. 8.8 Intraocular lens (IOL) scaffold for IOL exchange where a three-piece IOL is injected beneath the multifocal IOL that is then cut and removed. The three-piece IOL acts as a scaffold and prevents the posterior capsular damage. (These images are provided courtesy of Amar Agarwal.)

8.4.4 Intraocular Lens Scaffold

Narang et al described an innovative way to protect the posterior capsule during IOL exchange.[9] They advocate placing the new IOL under the original IOL first to act as a scaffold and to protect the posterior capsule while cutting the IOL optic. This technique can be particularly useful if laser posterior capsulotomy or other posterior capsule damage increases the possibility of IOL fragments falling posterior. Amar Agarwal agreed to share

▶ Fig. 8.8 where he has placed a three-piece IOL under an SPA multifocal before cutting it for removal.

8.5 Placing the New Intraocular Lens

8.5.1 Intraocular Lens Selection

The exchange does present an opportunity to modify the IOL power even when the indication for exchange was not refractive. It is important to discuss with the patient their refractive goals for the exchange. When the exchange is done for a refractive surprise, it is very important to retrace all calculations (particularly keratometric) and search for a reason for the refractive error. Often you can discover a missing piece of historical information (wore hard contact lenses prior to measurement) or a clerical error (transcription from device into formula) that clearly explains the refractive offset. The author's experience is that the new IOL power error is about 1.5 times more than the spectacle refraction error. For example, if the spectacle refractive error is a myopic surprise of 2 diopters, then the IOL power should be reduced by about 3 diopters.

8.5.2 Inserting the New Intraocular Lens

Other chapters will outline techniques for placing IOLs with limited capsular support. It is worthwhile to remind readers that while several interesting techniques exist for placing IOLs without capsular support (e.g., glued IOL, iris sutured IOL, etc.) there are no evidence that any of these techniques are superior to a well-placed AC IOL.[10] The preferred location for an IOL is either in the bag or a three-piece IOL with haptics in the sulcus and the optic prolapsed into the bag.[7]

The bag or sulcus should be prepared as usual with generous viscoelastic. The bag may require additional dissection as the IOLs have become free before the bag was completely open. If the bag is open completely and you have concerns for phimosis or mild zonular weakness, consider placement of a capsular tension ring (CTR). Centration is particularly important when placing a multifocal and a CTR may help keep a toric lens from rotating. The author likes to place a CTR and use traditional optic capture with the three-piece haptics in the sulcus and optic prolapsed back when he is concerned about weak zonules at present or in the future.

8.6 Conclusion

IOL exchange techniques are important to master for anterior segment surgeons. The indications for IOL exchange include implantation of the wrong power IOL, visual aberrations (e.g., halos, glare, and dysphotopsia), decentration/dislocation, opacification, and the UGH syndrome. In general, if the existing IOL can be secured or repositioned, that is preferable to IOL exchange. Explantation of the IOL from the capsular bag gets more difficult with time as the capsule becomes more adherent to the haptics. The IOL can be removed from the eye with a small incision by folding or cutting the IOL or it can simply be removed through a large incision.

8.7 Key Pearls

- The SPA is the most commonly exchanged IOL.
- Refractive IOL exchange occurs most commonly in the first 2 months.
- The most difficult part of an IOL exchange is freeing the haptics from the capsule.
- IOL exchange is made difficult by laser posterior capsulotomy.
- Consider using the scaffolding technique.

Videos

Video 8.1 Intraocular lens (IOL) exchange for broken haptic. The haptic of a three-piece IOL breaks after getting stuck in the plunger while being injected inside the eye. The IOL is rotated inside the AC and the other haptic is extruded from the corneal incision. The optic of the IOL is cut with MST Duet forceps and is explanted. A new three-piece IOL is then injected and is placed in the sulcus.

Video 8.2 Removal of opacified memory lens. The well-placed Intraocular lens (IOL) in the capsular bag is found to be opacified and necessitates an IOL exchange. Viscoat is injected with a 27-gauge needle between the IOL and the capsular margins to create a plane and remove the adhesions. As the haptics are firmly adherent to the capsular bag, they are cut at the optic–haptic junction on both sides. The IOL is eventually cut with IOL cutting scissors and is explanted. One of the haptic near corneal incision dislodges and is removed. Damage to the posterior capsule is noted and hence a three-piece foldable IOL is injected and placed into the sulcus. Anterior vitrectomy is done with the vitrectomy cutter and corneal sutures are taken to seal all the corneal incisions.

Video 8.3 Intraocular lens (IOL) exchange in phimotic capsule. Multiple relaxing incisions are placed on the phimotic anterior capsule to release the contractile force. The optic of the IOL is lifted and is manipulated in to the AC where it is cut and is explanted taking care not to drop the IOL piece into the vitreous cavity through the open posterior capsular yttrium aluminum garnet opening. Limited anterior vitrectomy is done and a three-piece IOL is injected and placed in to the sulcus.

References

[1] Mamalis N, Brubaker J, Davis D, Espandar L, Werner L. Complications of foldable intraocular lenses requiring explantation or secondary intervention–2007 survey update. J Cataract Refract Surg. 2008; 34(9):1584–1591

[2] Oetting TA. Uveitis-glaucoma-hyphema (UGH) syndrome. In: Randleman and Ahmed, eds. Intraocular Lens Surgery. New York, NY: Thieme Publisher; 2016:112–116

[3] Oetting TA. Explanting a posterior chamber intraocular lens. In: Agarwal A, Narang P, eds. Phacoemulsification. New Delhi: JayPee Highlights Medical Publisher; 2012:510–515

[4] Jin GJ, Crandall AS, Jones JJ. Intraocular lens exchange due to incorrect lens power. Ophthalmology. 2007; 114(3):417–424

[5] Davison JA. Positive and negative dysphotopsia in patients with acrylic intraocular lenses. J Cataract Refract Surg. 2004; 26:1346–1355

[6] Geneva II, Henderson BA. The complexities of negative dysphotopsia. Asia Pac J Ophthalmol (Phila). 2007; 6(4):364–371

[7] Kemp PS, Oetting TA. Stability and safety of MA50 intraocular lens placed in the sulcus. Eye (Lond). 2015; 29(11): 1438–1441

[8] Chang DF, Masket S, Miller KM, et al. ASCRS Cataract Clinical Committee. Complications of sulcus placement of single-piece acrylic intraocular lenses: recommendations for backup IOL implantation following posterior capsule rupture. J Cataract Refract Surg. 2009; 35(8):1445–1458

[9] Narang P, Steinert R, Little B, Agarwal A. Intraocular lens scaffold to facilitate intraocular lens exchange. J Cataract Refract Surg. 2014; 40(9):1403–1407

[10] Wagoner MD, Cox TA, Ariyasu RG, Jacobs DS, Karp CL, American Academy of Ophthalmology. Intraocular lens implantation in the absence of capsular support: a report by the American Academy of Ophthalmology. Ophthalmology. 2003; 110(4): 840–859

9 Piggyback Intraocular Lens

Johnny L. Gayton, Riley N. Sanders, and Val Nordin Sanders

Abstract

This chapter discusses the applicability of piggyback intraocular lenses (IOLs) including the method to calculate the IOL power of piggyback IOL and technique of implanting along with its advantages and disadvantages. The first primary piggyback IOL procedure was performed in 1992 in a nanophthalmic eye with a bag/sulcus technique. The procedure was modified to a bag/bag positioning for improved calculation outcome. This led to the postoperative complication of interlenticular opacity. In order to prevent this complication, the surgical technique returned to the original bag/sulcus IOL positioning. Due to improved IOL technology and calculations, primary piggyback procedure is rarely performed today. A secondary piggyback is much more common and is used to correct pseudophakic refractive error and dysphotopsia and to impart multifocality to pseudophakic patients.

Keywords: primary piggyback IOL, secondary piggyback IOL, effective lens position, refractive vergence formula, interlenticular opacification, pseudophakic refractive error

9.1 Origin

In 1992, a 31-year-old male presented with bilateral nanophthalmos desperate for help. He was employed by the state of Georgia and they had recently instituted uncorrected vision requirements of 20/60 for his position. His phakic spectacle prescription was $+19.25 + 0.25 \times 054$ right eye and $+19.52 + 0.25 \times 145$ left eye yielding best-corrected acuity of 20/50 bilaterally. He had mild nuclear sclerosis cataracts and refractive amblyopia compromising his vision. Axial length was measured at 15.80 mm right eye and 15.50 mm left eye. Keratometry was 46.50 sphere right eye and 46.50/47.25 in the left eye. Calculations were performed with the Sanders–Retzlaff–Kraff (SRK)/T formula indicating that a power of approximately 46 diopters would be needed to achieve a near plano postoperative refractive error. The dioptric range of IOL powers in the 1990s was limited to 10 to 30 diopter lenses to correct the normal axial length range. We were unable to find a manufacturer willing or able to produce such a high-powered lens for these nanophthalmic eyes.

After much thought, he was offered the possibility of inserting two intraocular lenses (IOLs); one three-piece plano convex lens in the bag with the plano side anterior and a second three-piece plano convex lens in the sulcus with the plano side posterior. After careful consideration and obtaining a second opinion, he agreed, as it was his only option. Initially a 25.0-diopter lens was implanted posteriorly and a 20.0-diopter lens anteriorly. The author seriously underestimated the power required, which led to the first IOL exchange of an anterior piggyback. The 20.0-diopter lens was exchanged for a 30.0-diopter lens and his resulting refraction was $+1.75 + 1.00 \times 95$. On the fellow eye, a 28.0-diopter lens implanted posteriorly and a 30.0-diopter lens anteriorly based largely on the results of his first eye. His refraction postoperatively was $-1.25 + 1.00 \times 60$ with best-corrected acuity of 20/50. His bilateral uncorrected visual acuity (VA) was 20/60 and he was able to continue working for the state until his retirement. The piggyback IOL procedure (▶ Fig. 9.1) was born.[1]

9.2 Refractive Considerations

As exemplified by the first case, the available IOL calculation formulas were not accurate for extremely long or short eyes. The available A-scan technology also was not as accurate in long or

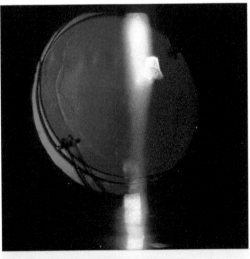

Fig. 9.1 Pristine postoperative piggyback lens.

short eyes. Measurement error in short axial length eyes results in a magnified refractive error. The leading IOL power consultants of the day (Holladay and Hill) began analyzing these early results and were able to make significant advances in available formulas. Dr. Jack Holladay and Dr. Jim Gills proposed that both lens be placed in the bag to improve power accuracy by controlling effective lens position. That was easily done since the bag is so much larger than the lens. The initial refractive outcome predictability improved dramatically with the double bag positioning and the advancement of IOL calculation software. The Holladay R IOL consultant created a module (refractive vergence formula) specifically for both primary and secondary piggyback procedures. Prior to the development of the Holladay R, 13% of the eyes receiving piggyback IOLs in our practice required secondary lens exchange to correct refractive error. It is still prudent to advise highly hyperopic patients of the possibility that an IOL exchange may be necessary, but it is an uncommon event today. It is also prudent to first operate on the nondominant eye so that the refractive results can be used to plan the dominant eye surgery for optimum outcome.

High-powered polymethyl methacrylate (PMMA) IOLs began to be more readily available toward the end of the 1990s, but piggybacking frequently was still a better option. The high-powered optics had significant aberrations and implantation required a larger incision. Due to difficulty in accurate measurements, lens exchange remained a possibility. When the centers of two piggyback IOLs are correctly aligned, they did provide better optical quality than a single high-power IOL. Additionally, it was safer to exchange a sulcus-positioned anterior lens than to exchange a capsule-positioned lens for refractive correction.

9.3 Surgical Complications

Inherent complications exist when operating on the hyperopic eye. The anterior chamber being smaller provides less working space. Positive vitreous pressure, posterior capsule rupture, iris prolapse, choroidal effusion, and aqueous misdirection have all been reported.[2] The corneal tunnel should be more anterior to lessen the likelihood of iris prolapse, and intravenous mannitol should be considered. The author makes a side port incision and temporal self-sealing corneal incision. The phacoemulsification wound is constructed so that the entry into the anterior chamber is made at least 2 mm anterior to

the limbus. The blade starts at the limbus, tunnels through the stroma, and enters through Descemet's membrane. This 2-mm tunnel is important in an effort to avoid iris prolapse. The capsulotomy should be made after filling the anterior chamber with a retentive viscoelastic. A less-than-full anterior chamber increases the risk of the capsular opening running radial. Radial extension can be particularly detrimental or disastrous in nanophthalmic eyes.

9.3.1 Long-Term Complications

The procedure gained popularity and began to be performed around the world. The technique seemed successful with complications generally related to residual refractive error for about 3 years. Douglas Koch told the author that he was seeing cases with cell growth between the lenses.[3] The author also began to see cases of interlenticular opacification (ILO), a complication that progressed from a hyperopic shift in refraction (shift of IOL position) to a significant loss of vision caused by opacity between the piggyback lenses (▶ Fig. 9.2) that was also noted by Dr. Joel Shugar.

Two of my patients had acrylic lenses explanted that were fused together (▶ Fig. 9.3). They were sent to Dr. David Apple, ophthalmic pathologist at Storm Eye Institute, for analysis. Histopathology of the opaque, membranelike material localized between the piggyback lenses identified retained regenerative cortex and proliferating lens epithelial cells, including bladder (Wedl's) cells. The composition replicated the pathologic process seen in posterior subcapsular cataracts and in the typical "pearl" form of posterior capsule opacification (PCO). Both sets of lenses with ILO analyzed seemed to be related to two PC IOLs being implanted in the capsular bag through a small capsulorhexis, with margins overlapping the optic edge of the anterior IOL for 360 degrees. Additionally, these lens sets were AcrySof material that demonstrates bioadhesion of the anterior surface of the front lens to the anterior capsule edge and of the posterior surface of the back lens to the posterior capsule.[4] The sealing of the space sequestered the lenses into a closed microenvironment. The cells, having nowhere else to go, accumulate in the interlenticular space.

9.4 Treatment of Interlenticular Opacity

Dr. Joel Shugar determined that the migration of the epithelial cells between the lenses only

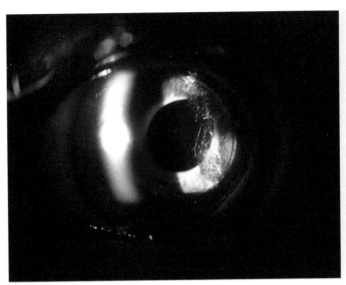

Fig. 9.2 Dense interlenticular membrane formation.

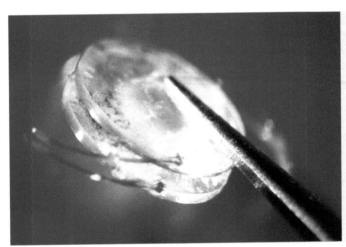

Fig. 9.3 Explanted intraocular lenses fused together. (This image is provided courtesy of David Apple, MD.)

occurred in piggybacks when the anterior capsule was on the anterior surface of the most anterior IOL 360 degrees.[5] We decided it was akin to grass growing through the cracks in concrete. The residual epithelial cells take the path of least resistance. When one lens was in the bag and one in the sulcus, the problem did not occur. When both lenses were in the bag, with a large capsulorhexis that was not in 360-degree contact with the anterior lens, the problem also did not happen. That led to prevention and treatment of ILO.

At the time, we had 167 cases of piggyback cases with 2 years or more of follow-up. Thirty-five ILO cases were identified and 23 were treated. Eleven eyes were treated with neodymium:yttrium aluminum garnet (Nd:YAG) laser of capsulorhexis and membrane (▸ Fig. 9.4, ▸ Fig. 9.5). Three eyes had YAG of capsulorhexis followed by aspiration of the interlenticular material and reposition of the anterior IOL into the sulcus.[6] Three eyes required both IOLs to be explanted. Three eyes were able to have the anterior IOL repositioned into the sulcus. Two eyes had an exchange of the anterior IOL. One eye had an exchange of the anterior IOL, excision of membrane, and lysis of synechiae. There was no definitive treatment as each was unique. Once we identified the cause of the complication, we were able to prophylactically treat eyes with YAG laser if the anterior capsule was on the surface of the most anterior lens to prevent development of ILO.

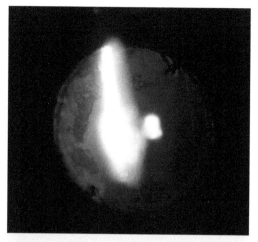

Fig. 9.4 Interlenticular opacity prior to yttrium aluminum garnet.

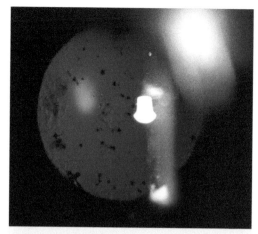

Fig. 9.5 Interlenticular opacity following yttrium aluminum garnet.

Although we had success treating ILO it is clearly preferable to avoid it altogether.

9.5 Prevention of Interlenticular Opacity

There are three options for the placement of piggyback lenses to avoid the development of ILO:
- Both posterior and anterior IOLs in the bag with a capsulorhexis larger than the anterior optic.
- Posterior IOL completely within the bag, anterior IOL haptics placed in the bag with the optic left outside the capsulorhexis.
- Posterior IOL in the capsular bag and anterior IOL in the sulcus. This is the most popular and the easiest to do. It is also the author's personal preference. This, along with careful cortical cleanup, prevents ILO.

After resolving the issue of ILO, piggybacks regained popularity primarily as a way to treat pseudophakic refractive error. Smaller refractive errors were generally treated with a three-piece silicone IOL. Larger errors were treated with smoothed edge three-piece acrylic lenses. Their higher index of refraction results in a thinner lens. Larger diopter silicone lenses were more likely to result in pupillary block. Pupillary block in piggybacks is treated by a peripheral iridotomy or removal of the piggyback. A smooth edge lens is preferable to prevent iris chaffing and pigment dispersion. Primary piggyback are rarely performed now because of improved accuracy of measurements and IOL calculations, intraprocedural aberrometry, and the availability of higher power lenses with improved optics. When they are performed, the anterior lens power should be chosen such that the power can be increased or decreased with an IOL exchange.

9.5.1 Secondary Piggyback Applications

Final refractive error of + 1.0 to −2.0 diopters is well tolerated by most patients, although cataract patients have much higher refractive expectations today. Moderate residual refractive errors of hyperopia, myopia, and astigmatism can be addressed with laser vision correction using laser in situ keratomileusis (LASIK), the small incision lenticule extraction (SMILE) procedure, or photorefractive keratectomy (PRK).[7] One retrospective study touted 93% of LASIK enhancements achieved spherical equivalent within 0.5 diopters of the target, 65% of secondary Piggyback IOLs were within 0.5 diopters of the target, and only 31% of IOL exchanges were within 0.5 diopters of target.[8] LASIK may be the most accurate method and reduces intraocular surgical risks, but not all patients are candidates for laser treatment. IOL-based procedures are a better choice for the ocular surface. An IOL exchange is rarely indicated exclusively for refractive error due to the inherent risks of the procedure. Higher amounts of pseudophakic error may be handled best with the insertion of a sulcus IOL.

Table 9.1 Considerations in correcting pseudophakic refractive error

Advantages of piggyback over laser vision correction	Advantages of piggyback over IOL exchange	Advantages of laser vision correction	Advantages of IOL exchange over piggyback
Less dry eye	More accurate	More accurate	Less risk of pupillary block
No flap complications	Easier to perform under topical anesthesia	No operating room (OR) fees	Less risk of pigment dispersion
Decreased risk of ocular surface issues	Less risk of capsular tear and vitreous loss complications	Minimal risk of intraocular complications	
Generally covered by insurance and less expensive equipment	Shorter OR time	Easier to treat astigmatism	
	Less risk of endothelial damage		

Abbreviations: IOL, intraocular lens.

Although the evolution of optical axial length biometry has greatly reduced axial length errors, patients with prior refractive surgery (PRK, radial keratotomy [RK], LASIK) or penetrating keratoplasty (PKP) have always been a challenge for accurate outcomes and are more likely to have residual refractive error. The use of intraoperative aberrometry (ORA System; Wave Tec Vision) has significantly reduced our pseudophakic enhancement rate (▶ Table 9.1). The secondary piggyback implant power can be calculated based on the current refraction so they can be more predictable than a lens exchange. The Holladay IIR software provides easy calculation although with hyperopia a close estimate may be calculated by multiplying 1.5 (residual refraction + desired; i.e., pseudophakic patient is a + 3.0 and the desired refraction is –0.5; 1.5 × 3.5 = + 5.25). When estimating for a myopic error, the formula is 1.2 (residual refraction + desired).[9]

The use of both multifocal and toric IOLs placed anteriorly has been gaining in popularity, especially in Europe. Anisometropia, astigmatism, and pseudophakic presbyopia are all being treated with secondary piggyback implantation. Currently, there are three companies manufacturing low-powered IOLs designed specifically for secondary sulcus implantation. These lenses are the Sulcoflex (Rayner Intraocular Lenses Ltd., East Sussex, UK), the Add-On (HumanOptics, Erlangen, Germany), and the 1stAdd-On (1stQ GmbH, Mannheim, Germany). Lens options include aspheric monofocal, multifocal, toric, and multifocal toric. The prospect of enhancing any pseudophakic patient with a refractive multifocal lens is exciting. The availability of multifocal lenses for piggybacking opens up a whole group of potential patients desiring to enhance their pseudophakic refractive outcome. The sulcus placed lens is less susceptible to decentration, but could be removed if a patient is bothered by aberrations from the multifocal optics.[10]

Piggyback IOLs have long been accepted as the treatment of choice for residual refractive error in PKP,[11] RK,[12] and LASIK patients. Compromised cornea tissue may be able to tolerate limbal relaxing incision (LRI) or PRK, but reaction to the treatment is far less predictable than a sulcus placed lens. Toric IOLs may also be a good option, especially if the intraoperative aberrometry is available. Another application for piggyback IOLs is in pediatric age group. When young children must have cataract surgery, the refractive error continues to shift toward myopia as the eye grows. A low-power IOL can be placed in the sulcus with the intention of removing it once the eye is fully grown and refraction is stable.[9,13]

9.6 Secondary Piggyback Complications

Optic capture of the secondary piggyback IOL by the iris can occur during the early postoperative period. This has been most commonly seen in patients receiving silicone myopic lenses. Most likely this is a function of the lens shape and thickness. Using a miotic immediately postoperatively and avoiding dilation the first few months after a secondary lens minimizes occurrence of this complication. Optic capture may be handled at the slit lamp using topical anesthesia. Use a 30-gauge needle inserted in a self-sealing fashion into the anterior chamber. Press the optic back into the posterior chamber, then instill topical pilocarpine until the pupil is smaller than the optic. Continue the pilocarpine postoperatively for a few months.[14]

9.7 Conclusion

In conclusion, the main reason for the development of the piggyback procedure is now by far its least common use. This is because of greater availability of a larger range of high-quality lens powers and more accurate methods of calculating lens powers. Secondary piggyback procedures are still common. In the United States, they are generally used to correct pseudophakic spherical refractive errors especially in those that are poor candidates for IOL exchange. Outside the United States, they are used to give patients multifocality, correct astigmatism, and correct spherical errors in pseudophakic patients. Hopefully, these improvements in piggyback lenses will one day be more widely available. Even though the piggyback technique is widely considered safe and effective, complications can and do occur. Proper preoperative evaluation and consent and close postoperative follow-up are essential to success.

9.8 Key Pearls

- Good surgical technique is essential for a successful primary and secondary piggyback IOL implantation.
- Secondary piggyback IOL implantation can be employed to address the higher refractive expectations of patients undergoing cataract surgery.
- Proper preoperative evaluation, consent, and follow-up are essential toward achieving a successful and an optimal surgical outcome.
- IOL power calculations in postrefractive surgery patients are harder to calculate and often these patients can be more demanding about their postcataract surgery refractive outcomes.
- ILO can usually be avoided and is amenable to treatment should it occur.

References

[1] Gayton JL, Sanders VN. Implanting two posterior chamber intraocular lenses in a case of microphthalmos. J Cataract Refract Surg. 1993; 19(6):776–777

[2] Utman SAK. Small eyes big problems: is cataract surgery the best option for the nanophthalmic eyes? J Coll Physicians Surg Pak. 2013; 23(9):653–656

[3] Jackson DW, Koch DD. Interlenticular opacification associated with asymmetric haptic fixation of the anterior intraocular lens. Am J Ophthalmol. 2003; 135(1):106–108

[4] Gayton JL, Apple DJ, Peng Q, et al. Interlenticular opacification: clinicopathological correlation of a complication of posterior chamber piggyback intraocular lenses. J Cataract Refract Surg. 2000; 26(3):330–336

[5] Shugar JK, Keeler S. Interpseudophakos intraocular lens surface opacification as a late complication of piggyback acrylic posterior chamber lens implantation. J Cataract Refract Surg. 2000; 26(3):448–455

[6] Gayton JL, Van der Karr M, Sanders V. Neodymium:YAG treatment of interlenticular opacification in a secondary piggyback case. J Cataract Refract Surg. 2001; 27(9):1511–1513

[7] Artola A, Ayala M, Claramonte P, Perez-Santonja J, Alió JL. Photorefractive keratectomy for residual myopia after cataract surgery. J Cataract Refract Surg. 1999; 25: 1456–1460

[8] Fernandez-Buenaga R, Allio JL, Perez Ardoy AL, Pinill-Cortes L. Resolving refractive error after cataract surgery: IOL exchange, piggyback lens, or LASIK. J Cataract Refract Surg. 2013; 10:676–683

[9] Rubenstein J. Piggyback IOLs for residual refractive error after cataract surgery. Cataract Refract Surg Today. 2012. Available at: https://crstoday.com/articles/2012-aug/piggyback-iols-for-residual-refractive-error-after-cataract-surgery

[10] Hoffman R. Sulcoflex IOLs Offer future options for refractive enhancements. 2010. Available at: https://www.eyeworld.org/

[11] Paul RA, Chew HF, Singal N, Rootman DS, Slomovic AR. Piggyback intraocular lens implantation to correct myopic pseudophakic refractive error after penetrating keratoplasty. J Cataract Refract Surg. 2004; 30(4):821–825

[12] Hill WE. Refractive enhancement with piggybacking IOLs. In: Chang DF, ed. Mastering Refractive IOLs: The Art and Science. Thorofare, NJ: Slack Inc; 2008;792–793

[13] Boisvert C, Beverly DT, McClatchey SK. Theoretical strategy for choosing piggyback intraocular lens powers in young children. J AAPOS. 2009; 13(6):555–557

[14] Gayton JL, Sanders V, Van Der Karr M. Pupillary capture of the optic in secondary piggyback implantation. J Cataract Refract Surg. 2001; 27(9):1514–1515

10 Toric Intraocular Lens

Eric Clayton Amesbury and Kevin M. Miller

Abstract

Cataract surgeons should be prepared to deal with suboptimal refractive results after phacoemulsification with toric intraocular lens implantation. Tips for avoiding and dealing with suboptimal results are discussed in this chapter. Clinical examples are provided for illustration.

Keywords: lenses, intraocular lens implantation, astigmatism, phacoemulsification, cataract, cataract extraction, refractive surgical procedures, cornea, pseudophakia

10.1 Introduction

Clinically significant corneal astigmatism is commonly found in a significant proportion of cataract surgery patients. Astigmatism correction at the time of cataract surgery can improve postoperative visual outcomes and reduce dependence on corrective lenses. In addition to other treatment options, including operating on the steep axis and peripheral corneal relaxing incisions (PCRIs), toric intraocular lens (IOL) implantation can achieve excellent astigmatic correction. Cataract surgeons should be prepared to deal with suboptimal refractive results after toric IOL implantation. Tips for avoiding and dealing with suboptimal results are discussed in this chapter. Clinical examples are provided for illustration.

10.2 Preoperative Planning

Preoperative planning for toric IOL implantation requires evaluation for preexisting corneal conditions, which may affect keratometry and refractive outcomes. A partial list includes dry eye, pterygium, Fuchs' dystrophy, Salzmann's nodular degeneration, keratoconus, prior corneal transplantation, prior scleral buckling, and epithelial basement membrane dystrophy. Identification and treatment of these conditions followed by adequate time for stabilization of the cornea and ocular surface are required before biometry and IOL selection are completed.

Spherical IOL power calculation inaccuracy can negatively impact the refractive outcome of toric IOL implantation. Optical biometry using partial coherence interferometry has become increasingly accurate for axial length determination, but keratometric assumptions inherent in most devices are not always accurate for determining total corneal power. The accuracy of these devices is especially reduced for eyes that have undergone corneal refractive surgery. Keratoconus and other corneal ectasias will also impact the accuracy of biometry. Additionally, eyes with irregular astigmatism may not be amenable to treatment with toric IOLs.

Corneal topography and tomography should be obtained to identify these conditions and act as an additional check on corneal power estimation by optical biometry. Manual keratometry may also be useful for comparison, looking for consistency across multiple measurements before completing calculations and IOL selection. As with keratometry, axial length measurement methods can introduce error. Optical biometry cannot penetrate dense cataracts and ultrasonography may occasionally be needed. Corneal compression during contact ultrasonic measurements will provide a falsely shorter axial length, which can be avoided with the immersion technique. Excessively long or short eyes additionally challenge the accurate calculation of IOL power. Long eyes (> 26 mm) need an adjustment factor when using "third-generation" formulas. Alternatively, formulas requiring measurements besides axial length and keratometry, such as anterior chamber depth, can increase accuracy. The Sanders–Retzlaff–Kraff (SRK)/T, Haigis, Barrett Universal II, Holladay 2, and Olsen formulas offer the best prediction of refractive results for axial length greater than 26 mm and IOL power 6.0 diopters or higher.[1] Similarly, for short eyes (< 20 mm) the Hoffer Q appears to be more accurate for IOL calculation than SRK/T, but further study is needed. Kapamajian and Miller have proposed a correction for eyes that require negative power IOLs.[2]

10.3 Toric Power Calculation

Early toric IOL calculators have proven to be less accurate than previously thought. Some of the errors come from ignoring the vertex effect on toric IOL power calculation. Toric IOL calculation using the Barrett toric IOL calculator, or Abulafia–Koch adjustment added to the Alcon or Holladay calculator, using vector analysis, reportedly achieves a result of 77 to 78% within ± 0.50 diopter cylinder predicted.[3] Without directly measuring posterior corneal astigmatism, it is common to overestimate with-the-rule (WTR) and underestimate against-the-rule (ATR) astigmatism.[4] Even when compensating for the effect of the posterior cornea, we recommend undertreating WTR astigmatism and overtreating ATR when planning toric IOL implantation. A residual astigmatism of 0.3-diopter WTR postoperatively allows for some age-related postoperative drift in astigmatism without negative consequences on uncorrected visual acuity. Accurately estimating surgically induced astigmatism (SIA) is important for calculations. We recommend using 0.4 diopter of SIA for an incision width of 2.4 to 2.75 mm, and reducing the estimate for a smaller incision.

10.4 Surgical Considerations

During surgery, compensation for cyclotorsion is achieved with a single preoperative limbal mark at the 6 o'clock position or two marks at the 3 and 9 o'clock positions, placed with the patient sitting upright. Intraoperative guidance systems (Alcon Laboratories Verion and ORA, Zeiss CALLISTO Eye, Clarity Medical Systems HOLOS IntraOp, and True-Vision Systems TrueGuide), which compare anatomic recognition to a reference image, are also useful adjuncts. Digital platforms have additional features such as intraoperative guides for PCRI and surgical incision placement. Some are capable of intraoperative aberrometry. When marking by hand, the target meridian for toric IOL alignment is confirmed and marked intraoperatively with the aid of a corneal gauge. Mean IOL alignment error using this method was found to be approximately 5% in one study.[5] To minimize alignment error, care must be taken to avoid letting marks spread and to carefully align the visual axis of the eye with the surgical microscope view. After implantation and rotation of the IOL to within a few degrees of the target meridian, meticulous removal of viscoelastic material reduces the likelihood of IOL rotation postoperatively. The surgeon should not let the anterior chamber shallow postoperatively as this may cause unwanted IOL rotation. A final check of the IOL alignment with the target meridian should be done as the last step. When a pupil expansion device is removed, iris constriction can limit visualization of the IOL orientation. Thus, a small pupil may be considered a minor relative contraindication to implantation of a toric IOL. Patients should be cautioned against touching or rubbing the eye after surgery to avoid rotating the axis of the IOL. Capsule tension ring implantation may lessen the likelihood of toric IOL rotation in large myopic eyes with large capsular bags.

10.5 Suboptimal Outcomes

The etiology of a suboptimal refractive outcome should be identified, if possible, prior to fellow eye surgery. This process begins with a thorough examination. Besides preexisting ocular comorbidity, common postoperative complications such as excessive inflammation and delayed wound healing should be ruled out. Posterior capsule opacification and cystoid macular edema should be identified and treated if present.

Lenticular astigmatism may contribute to "whole-eye" astigmatism and be reflected in the preoperative manifest refraction. Preoperative astigmatism planning, however, considers only preoperative corneal astigmatism. Postoperatively, barring a decentered or tilted IOL, or toric IOL implantation, there should be no unwanted lenticular astigmatism.

IOL manufacturers have an allowable spherical power error range of ±0.25 diopters, which, when combined with another error, could be visually significant. IOL tilt, decentration, and a lens position within the eye other than that anticipated by IOL calculations may impact the effective toric power of the IOL. A consistently round and centered capsulorrhexis, sized to cover the anterior edge of the IOL, is considered ideal and provides more reliable outcome data upon which to base a surgeon adjustment factor. As mentioned previously, using a vector analysis toric IOL calculator such as the Barrett online calculator is helpful.

Assuming that the target meridian for toric IOL alignment is calculated and marked correctly, postoperative IOL rotation should be ruled out. This is done with a dilated pupil at the slit lamp biomicroscope, noting the orientation of the alignment marks on the toric IOL with the head perfectly straight. A reticule attached to the slit lamp, or aberrometry, can aid identification of the axis of the implant. If these methods are not available, using the clock hour of the implant alignment provides a fair estimate of the toric axis. Rotation in the early postoperative period was especially problematic with early plate haptic toric IOLs, especially those with a short haptic length. They were slippery and tended to find the long axis of the capsular bag. Rotations are less frequent with open loop haptic IOL designs. Opinions vary in the literature as to how much cylinder correction is lost from a misaligned toric IOL, but it is generally accepted that for every degree of misalignment the estimated reduction in astigmatic correction at the cornea plane is 3%.

10.6 Managing Residual Refractive Error

Nonsurgical treatment options include corrective spectacles or soft toric contact lenses. Rigid contact lenses are not recommended as they unmask lenticular astigmatism.

IOL repositioning should be considered on a case-by-case basis. The magnitude of cylinder power is important. A toric IOL with a low cylinder correction at the corneal plane, when misaligned less than 5 degrees, will yield limited potential benefit if repositioned. Surgical reintervention must be weighed against the risks of the intraocular procedure. For higher power toric IOLs, even a small misalignment can reduce visual outcome significantly, and may warrant repositioning.

Surgical options for correction of suboptimal refractive results after toric IOL implantation include corneal refractive surgery such as relaxing incisions, laser in situ keratomileusis (LASIK), and photorefractive keratectomy (PRK); IOL repositioning; IOL exchange; and piggyback IOL implantation. The status of the lens capsule is important when considering surgical correction of residual astigmatism. Corneal refractive surgery does not depend on an intact capsule. Small residual refractive errors are effectively corrected with laser refractive surgery. Before proceeding, we recommend waiting 3 months for refractive stability. PCRIs can correct mixed astigmatism up to 2.5-diopter cylinder and can be done with manual blades or a femtosecond laser. Preplaced femtosecond stromal incisions can be selectively opened during or after surgery to titrate astigmatic correction.[6]

Larger refractive errors may be treated by IOL repositioning or exchange. This approach requires an intact capsular bag and is best performed early in the postoperative period to avoid capsular fibrosis. If anterior capsule polishing is performed at the time of surgery, it will result in less fibrosis and easier IOL manipulation. Toric IOL repositioning can be considered if the residual spherical equivalent (SE) refractive error is less than 0.5 diopters. One should attempt to reopen the original incision. The goal is to align the toric IOL with the steep axis of postoperative corneal cylinder, not the original target meridian from preoperative calculations. Toric IOL exchange is reserved for SE errors greater than 0.5 diopters or when there is a problem with the lens itself. A piggyback IOL can be considered for treating simple myopic or hyperopic refractive errors greater than 1 diopter. The procedure carries less risk of incorrect IOL power, capsule rupture, vitreous loss, and cystoid macular edema as opposed to IOL exchange, balanced against risks including pigment dispersion. We recommend a three-piece, rounded-edge silicone IOL such as the Staar AQ5010V implanted in the ciliary sulcus to avoid interlenticular fibrosis and late hyperopic shift. Piggyback IOL implantation can reduce the effective power of the primary IOL if the zonules are loose, resulting in a surprise hyperopic shift.

10.7 Clinical Examples

To wrap up this chapter, we present three patients who had postoperative problems following toric IOL implantation. Each presented with a unique set of circumstances and each required a different management approach.

10.7.1 Case 1: Photorefractive Keratectomy Enhancement

This patient had a history of myopic LASIK, followed by cataract extraction with toric IOL implantation, in both eyes. Neodymium:yttrium aluminum garnet (Nd:YAG) laser capsulotomies had been performed several months before initial evaluation. At the time of presentation, the patient complained of blurred vision in both eyes. Examination revealed small central posterior capsule openings in both eyes, opacified peripheral capsules, and a few pits on the lens in the right eye. Laser capsulotomy enlargements were performed in both eyes and resulted in much improved glare sensitivity and nighttime vision. At a follow-up visit, the patient expressed an interest in undergoing a refractive enhancement to improve the uncorrected distance visual acuity (UDVA). Examination revealed UDVA of 20/30 in the right eye and 20/25 in the left eye. The manifest refractive error of the right eye was –1.75 + 0.50 × 144, resulting in corrected distance visual acuity (CDVA) of 20/15 –1. Manifest refraction

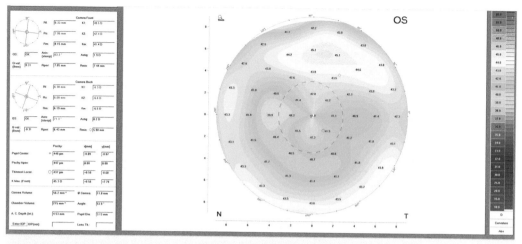

Fig. 10.1 Corneal topography before photorefractive keratectomy enhancement.

of the left eye was −1.75 + 0.50 × 116, resulting in CDVA of 20/20 + 2. Pachymetry measurements were 440 and 486 μm, respectively. Preoperative Pentacam corneal topography is shown in ▶ Fig. 10.1. After discussing the options, we decided to proceed with PRK enhancement of the left eye to improve UDVA. If the patient could not adjust to the resulting monovision, we would perform the same procedure on the right eye sometime afterward to balance the two eyes. One month after PRK, the patient was satisfied with the outcome and comfortable with the resulting monovision. UDVA was 20/40 in the right eye and 20/15 in the left eye. The manifest refraction of the left eye was −0.25 + 0.50 × 030, resulting in unchanged CDVA of 20/15.

Comment: Given the open posterior capsules in this case, IOL exchange is not a good option. Not only would it place the patient at significant risk of retinal detachment and cystoid macular edema, but also the replacement lens could not be toric, so the patient would experience an improved spherical error but a worsened cylinder error. A LASIK enhancement would be easy to perform, even 15 years after the original procedure, but the risk of postoperative epithelial ingrowth would be high and the procedure would thin the posterior stromal bed even further, risking ectasia. PRK is the most reasonable option as it reduces the myopic error without compromising toric correction and preserves the biomechanical strength of the cornea.

10.7.2 Case 2: Toric Intraocular Lens Rotation

This patient presented with a history notable for traumatic retinal detachment repair by scleral buckle in the right eye. Subsequent scleral buckle removal or prism glasses did not resolve residual strabismus and diplopia. The patient was less troubled by double vision over time as a cataract developed. At the time of presentation, CDVA of the right eye was 20/400 with moderate right exotropia. Manifest refraction was −5.25 sphere for the right eye and −4.75 + 1.75 × 097 for the left eye. Slit-lamp biomicroscopy revealed a 4 + brunescent cataract in the right eye with mild phacodonesis and a poorly dilated pupil. Partial coherence interferometry could not be performed because the cataract was too dense, so axial length was determined by A-scan ultrasonography. Pentacam corneal topography revealed 3.3 diopters of anterior corneal astigmatism at 98.6 degrees in the right eye (▶ Fig. 10.2) and 3.5 diopters of total corneal astigmatism at 99.5 degrees. Alcon toric lens power calculation called for an SN6AT8 lens at 98 degrees (▶ Fig. 10.3). Complex phacoemulsification and toric IOL implantation were performed on the right eye, with an emmetropic refractive goal. Three weeks after surgery, UDVA was 20/80 + 2 with manifest refraction of −2.25 + 2.25 × 142, resulting in CDVA of 20/25. Corneal topography was essentially unchanged. Examination revealed that the toric optic was oriented at 80 degrees instead of 98 degrees. Because the anisometropia

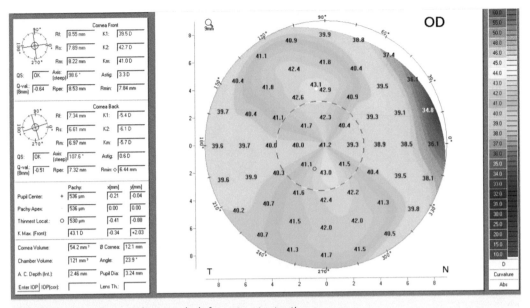

Fig. 10.2 Preoperative corneal topography before cataract extraction.

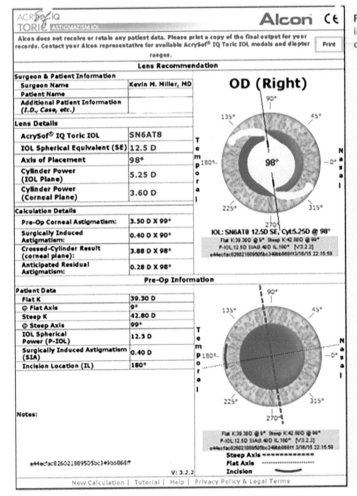

Fig. 10.3 Preoperative Alcon toric intraocular lens calculation before cataract extraction.

would have been made worse if the −1.125 diopter (SE) myopic refractive error had been corrected by lens exchange, we made the decision to rotate the toric IOL to the correct axis. One month after repositioning, UDVA was 20/30 −2. Manifest refraction of the right eye was −1.00 + 0.75 × 010 with CDVA of 20/25 + 2. Optical coherence tomography testing of the macula revealed normal anatomy. The left eye UDVA was 20/100 −2, and the patient elected to undergo cataract extraction with toric IOL implantation for that eye, resulting in UDVA of 20/15 −1. The patient was happy with mild monovision and not bothered by diplopia from the exotropia of the right eye.

Comment: Toric lens rotation is a reasonable surgical alternative if it can be performed relatively soon after cataract surgery, the capsular bag is intact, and no alteration is needed in the spherical power of the IOL or the power of the toric component of the optic. An alternative is corneal relaxing incisions to rotate the axis of corneal cylinder to align with the axis of the toric cylinder. Corneal refractive surgery could also be performed, but it would have to be a mixed astigmatism correction, which is not ideal. Relaxing incisions or corneal refractive surgery would have been more reasonable choices if the posterior capsule were already open.

10.7.3 Case 3: Toric Intraocular Lens Exchange

The patient presented with blurred vision in both eyes, worse in the right eye. There was no known significant ocular history. CDVAs were 20/40 for the right eye and 20/25 for the left eye, with manifest refraction of + 0.25 + 2.50 × 005 in the right eye and + 0.25 + 3.25 × 175 in the left eye. Mixed age-related cataracts were observed on slit-lamp biomicroscopy in both eyes. Pentacam corneal topography revealed previously undetected keratoconus with slightly asymmetric bowtie astigmatism in both eyes (▶ Fig. 10.4, ▶ Fig. 10.5). There was no skewing of the axis in either eye. Central corneal thickness was 473 μm for the right eye and 433 μm for the left eye. The patient declined the option of a rigid contact lens and the corneal astigmatism was only mildly asymmetric, so we decided to implant toric IOLs in both eyes. Alcon toric planning called for an SN6AT7 in the right eye (▶ Fig. 10.6). UDVA was 20/30 the day after surgery. Two weeks after surgery, the patient complained of decreased vision. UDVA had declined to 20/60 with manifest refraction of −3.00 + 3.25 × 138, resulting in DCVA of 20/25 + 1. On examination, the toric marks on the lens were oriented at 108 degrees, compared to the goal meridian 130 degrees. After further observation, UDVA settled to 20/80 −2 with unchanged

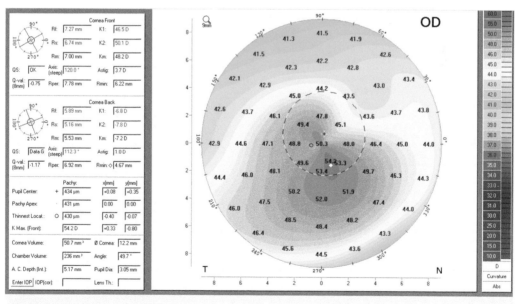

Fig. 10.4 Corneal topography, right eye.

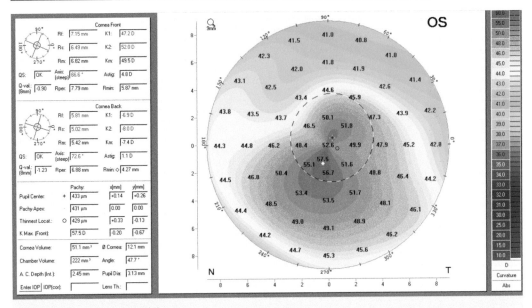

Fig. 10.5 Corneal topography, left eye.

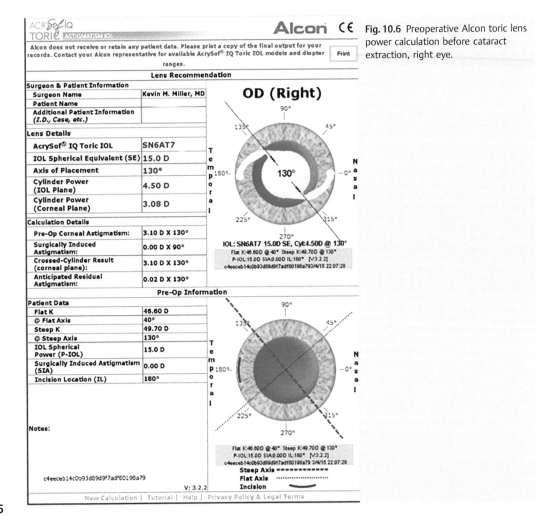

Fig. 10.6 Preoperative Alcon toric lens power calculation before cataract extraction, right eye.

Berdahl & Hardten Toric IOL Calculator Results

Physician Name:
Physician Email:

Patient Name:
Patient Eye: Right Eye
Originally Calculated IOL Axis (Degrees): 118

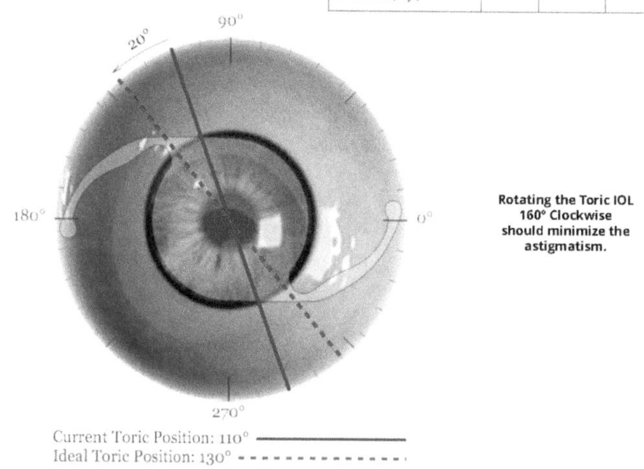

Fig. 10.7 Berdahl & Hardten Astigmatism Fix calculation before toric IOL exchange, right eye.

Entered Data

	Sphere	Cylinder (plus power)	Axis (Deg)
Toric Lens		3.08	110
Current Refraction (+cyl)	-2.75	4.00	145

Calculated Results

	Sphere	Cylinder (plus power)	Axis (Deg)
Ideal Position of the Toric		3.08	130
Expected Residual Refraction (+cyl)	-2.12	2.74	130

Rotating the Toric IOL 160° Clockwise should minimize the astigmatism.

Current Toric Position: 110° ————
Ideal Toric Position: 130° - - - - - - - - - - - - - -

refraction. Rather than rotate the lens, we elected to exchange it to correct the small myopic refractive error in addition to the increased postoperative corneal astigmatism. The Berdahl & Hardten Astigmatism Fix calculation is shown in ▶ Fig. 10.7. The Barrett toric calculation is shown in ▶ Fig. 10.8. Toric lens exchange was performed. The old lens was refolded inside the eye over a cyclodialysis spatula and removed through a slightly enlarged phacoemulsification incision. An Alcon SN6AT9 replacement IOL was implanted and oriented at 130 degrees. Left eye cataract surgery with toric IOL implantation was performed resulting in UDVA 20/30 −1 with some residual cylinder, but the patient was happy with the result. Nd:YAG laser capsulotomy was subsequently performed. One month after the lens exchange in the right eye, final UDVAs were 20/25 + 1 in the right eye and 20/25 + 2 in the left eye. The manifest refractive errors were minimal and required glasses only for reading at near.

Comment: Surgical options for correcting the postoperative refractive error of the right eye in this case include laser refractive surgery and IOL exchange. IOL rotation cannot reduce the spherical or astigmatic errors of the eye. Given that the cataract surgery was relatively recent, the capsular bag was intact, and the patient's cornea was relatively thin from keratoconus, toric IOL exchange was the procedure of choice.

10.8 Key Pearls

- Toric IOLs help correct regular corneal astigmatism and not an irregular astigmatism. Patients with irregular astigmatism do not fare well with toric IOL placement.
- It is extremely crucial to differentiate lenticular astigmatism from corneal astigmatism.
- Surgically induced astigmatism should be taken into consideration while calculating the extent of astigmatism that can be corrected.
- Precise reference marking of the cornea should be done before the surgical procedure with the patient in an upright sitting position.
- Ophthalmic viscosurgical device must be completely removed from the eye at the end of the procedure and the IOL alignment should be checked.

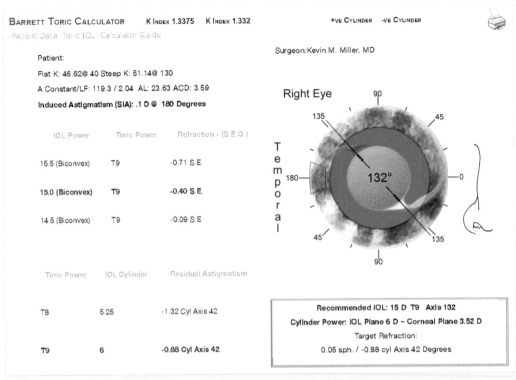

Fig. 10.8 Barrett toric intraocular lens (IOL) calculation before toric IOL exchange, right eye.

References

[1] Abulafia A, Barrett GD, Rotenberg M, et al. Intraocular lens power calculation for eyes with an axial length greater than 26.0 mm: comparison of formulas and methods. J Cataract Refract Surg. 2015; 41(3):548–556

[2] Kapamajian MA, Miller KM. Efficacy and safety of cataract extraction with negative power intraocular lens implantation. Open Ophthalmol J. 2008; 2:15–19

[3] Abulafia A, Koch DD, Wang L, et al. New regression formula for toric intraocular lens calculations. J Cataract Refract Surg. 2016; 42(5):663–671

[4] Koch DD, Jenkins RB, Weikert MP, Yeu E, Wang L. Correcting astigmatism with toric intraocular lenses: effect of posterior corneal astigmatism. J Cataract Refract Surg. 2013; 39(12): 1803–1809

[5] Visser N, Berendschot TTJM, Bauer NJC, Jurich J, Kersting O, Nuijts RMMA. Accuracy of toric intraocular lens implantation in cataract and refractive surgery. J Cataract Refract Surg. 2011; 37(8):1394–1402

[6] Rückl T, Dexl AK, Bachernegg A, et al. Femtosecond laser-assisted intrastromal arcuate keratotomy to reduce corneal astigmatism. J Cataract Refract Surg. 2013; 39(4):528–538

11 Premium Intraocular Lenses and Associated Problems

Elizabeth Yeu and Mario J. Rojas

Abstract

This chapter focuses on premium and advanced technology presbyopia-correcting intraocular lenses (PCIOLs) highlighting ways to maximize surgical outcomes. The various IOL platforms and options are discussed, including accommodating, multifocal, extended depth of focus (EDOF) IOLs and their presbyopia-correcting toric IOL options. An overview of their mechanisms, along with their limitations based on their optical properties, is reviewed, with a review of the literature on the performance of the IOLs. An ounce of prevention is worth more than a pound of cure, and this holds evermore true for the patient selection and preparation process with PCIOLs. Preoperatively, setting appropriate expectations, sufficient chair time, and patient-specific characteristics (height, near vision needs) are as important as accurate diagnostics, a healthy macula, and ocular surface stabilization. The chapter hones in on postoperative evaluation and management of the surprise result or the less-than-satisfied postoperative patient, highlighting the various tools and treatment options available to maximize patient outcomes and satisfaction. The more common causes of pseudophakic dissatisfaction include a missed refractive target, ocular surface disease and subjective concerns thereof, posterior capsular opacification, and IOL-related issues. Various diagnostic and treatment approaches are reviewed, including corneal refractive enhancement options, when to consider an IOL exchange, and piggyback IOL options.

Keywords: premium IOL, multifocal IOL, EDOF IOL, accommodating IOL, presbyopia-correcting IOL, management of postoperative pseudophakic surprise

11.1 Introduction

The greatest challenge that a surgeon meets with multifocal intraocular lens (MFIOL) is the management of a patient with suboptimal visual acuity or management of a patient with a poor quality of vision despite having 20/20 vision on Snellen's chart. The nuances and problems associated with multifocal, accommodative, and other premium IOLs and the need to meet the never-ending demands of patients are the highlights of the chapter and will be discussed in detail.

11.2 Presbyopia-Correcting Intraocular Lenses

Presbyopia is an age-related condition, which gradually decreases an individual's ability to accommodate to a near object. This condition affects the majority of the aging population, and worsens with age. Cataract surgery is not only an excellent opportunity to maximize an individual's best-corrected vision, but also offers the possibility to fulfill the needs our patients have for uncorrected distance, intermediate, and near vision. Our IOL options and technology continue to improve, and with the increased options comes the ability to maximize our patients' uncorrected range of vision after cataract surgery. Understanding the mechanisms of each of the premium IOLs on the market, and how they manipulate incoming light, is invaluable to addressing each patient's needs for the best premium IOL selection.

Before diving into the benefits and limitations of various premium IOLs, it is important to note a certain level of dissatisfaction with monofocal IOLs. Several studies have shown monofocal control groups to reveal a few noteworthy subjective outcomes. It has been reported that 3 to 8% of patients implanted with monofocal IOLs were found to have enough uncorrected near vision to read newspaper print. At the other end of the spectrum, results from several studies have reported incidence of positive dysphotopsias, such as glare, halos, and the night vision symptoms, despite not being graded as severe. Negative dysphotopsia is also a well-recognized and clinically frustrating photopsia, which occurs in patients who have received monofocal IOLs, and this manifests as temporal "crescent" of "missing vision."[1] There are two groups of presbyopia-correcting IOLs that are more widely utilized: accommodative and MFIOLs. While there are certain side effects and complications that are unique to their respective IOL designs, the overall approach to the assessment and management of the less-than-satisfied postoperative patient is a similar one.

Accommodative IOLs have been on the market for over 10 years, and have embraced the philosophy drawn out by the Helmholtz model of accommodation. The design and purpose of accommodative IOLs, such as the Crystalens, Tetraflex, and the 1 Component Unit (1CU) was to make an IOL pliable enough to bend and be displaced forward as the eye responds to its natural tendency to accommodate. The displacement forward would theoretically allow a pseudoaccommodative state, increasing the effective power of the lens, to address intermediate and near vision, and Heatley et al did an excellent job, mathematically demonstrating how 1-diopter accommodation could be achieved with an increase in effective pseudoaccommodation.[2] A recent study using anterior segment imaging demonstrated axial shifts of the accommodating IOL were small, and in many cases the lens shifted backward on accommodative effort.[3] A similar study used ultrasonic biomicroscopy (UBM) technology and showed a mean accommodative amplitude of 0.44 ± 0.24 diopters, which was calculated to be a range of accommodation approximately 0.25 to 0.75 diopters.[4] This may clinically translate to variable amounts of near vision postoperatively, and a patient experiencing a lack of adequate pseudoaccommodative amplitude could certainly lead to dissatisfaction. Such inconsistent near vision outcomes were demonstrated by a large meta-analysis that reviewed four randomized clinical trials (RCTs) with the 1CU and the AT-45 IOLs, where considerable heterogeneity of effect was seen, with near vision ranging from 1.3 to 6 Jaeger units and 0.12 logMAR improvement.[5]

The shear design of accommodative IOLs does limit the degree of dysphotopsias, such as glare, halos, or starbursts. Takakura et al reported a large meta-analysis that reviewed two RCTs, each demonstrating no significant difference in glare or contrast sensitivity.[6] With such a sound optical system, and toric options available, accommodative IOLs are excellent options for the patients who value uncorrected distance visual acuity (UCDVA) and who understand their uncorrected near visual acuity (UCNVA) may be limited and who do not want to risk having other secondary optical dysphotopsias. From the surgeon's perspective, a low incidence of posterior capsule opacification and capsular fibrosis is crucial, as both can be a long-term detrimental factor for near vision needs in accommodating IOLs, not to mention what is known as Z syndrome. In Z syndrome, the capsule contracts and causes compression along the haptic–optic axis, resulting in asymmetric folding. The asymmetric vaulting of the lens resembles a Z, and results in tilting of the optic, which can lead to coma aberration, increased myopia, and increased astigmatism. For subtle cases and a high index of suspicion, diagnostic equipment, such as the NIDEK OPD III or iTrace, may help determine IOL tilt or Z syndrome. Capsular bag rigidity limits axial movement of the IOLs and therefore reduces accommodative capacity. An early posterior capsulotomy after postoperative 1 month has been advocated to prevent unwanted complications from capsular fibrosis. If a Z syndrome does occur, strategic neodymium:yttrium aluminum garnet (Nd:YAG) laser dissection of the anterior and/or posterior capsule, or even placement of a capsular tension ring, can effectively alleviate this complication.[7]

Regarding MFIOL technology, until 2005, they were designed with strictly refractive technology. This design had its limitations, and along came the first diffractive lenses, which have continually evolved. Complaints of glare and halos with night driving with earlier iterations were common, and this has continued to improve with refinements such as aspheric transitions between optical zones.[8] Regardless of the dysphotopsia, UCNVA became attainable. Fortunately, newer generation low-add multifocals have led to decreased unwanted night vision dysphotopsias[9,10] and greater quality of overall vision, and have improved intermediate visual acuity. Several studies have shown less dysphotopsias, in the low adds compared to their respective 4.0 add models.[11] The subjective complaints of MFIOLs are of no surprise, as several objective studies have predicted these phenomena. There is overall significantly improved postoperative satisfaction in patients with +2.75 or +3.25 diopter add than those with a +4.00 diopter add.[12]

The low-add multifocals can effectively provide both intermediate and near vision needs, and patients with the lowest add MFIOL can achieve significant spectacle independence.[9,10,13] Combining different strength MFIOLs can lead to greater near vision satisfaction. Mastropasqua et al reported a prospective nonrandomized single-blind observational study where patients received either the Restor SN6AD1 + 3.0 diopter lens or the Restor SV25T0 + 2.5 diopter lens in either eye, or one of each. The National Eye Institute's Refractive Error Quality of Life instrument (NEI RQL42) questionnaire showed that combining the different IOLs produced better results in terms of expectations and activity limitations, while contrast sensitivity showed no difference between groups.[12]

With any MFIOL, understanding our patient's needs and requirement for near vision versus intermediate vision can be the difference between a 20/20 happy patient and a 20/20 unhappy patient.

A recent retrospective study reviewed a large group of patients who presented after either MFIOL implantation or an accommodative IOL placement. The chief complaint of 29 (59%) patients was blurry vision, both for distance and near; this was seen in 50 eyes (68%).[14] An in vitro study by Vega and colleagues demonstrated that various MFIOLs could still lead to unwanted dysphotopsias. The SV25T0 + 2.5 had smaller but more intense halo formation than the ZKB00 + 2.75. The SV25T0 + 2.5 also showed a deceased halo size, but increase in intensity with an increase in pupil size from 3.0 to 4.5 mm (▶ Fig. 11.1).[15,16]

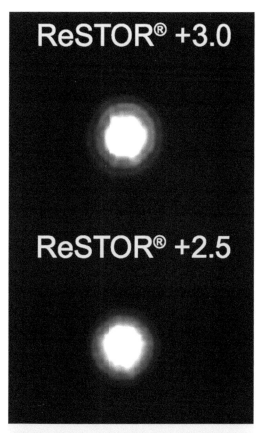

Fig. 11.1 This is an in vitro simulation of oncoming headlights in a 5-mm pupil of two multifocal intraocular lenses (MFIOLs) with different add-ons. As demonstrated by the images, the IOL with the stronger add power, ReSTOR 3.0, has a wider halo and glare profile than the weaker low-add ReSTOR 2.5.

11.3 Extended Depth of Focus Intraocular Lens

The current generation of diffractive IOLs fall under the spectrum of extended depth of focus (EDOF). The technology is based on a modification to the traditional MFIOLs. The TECNIS Symfony is an example, and is a biconvex and pupil-independent diffractive IOL, and combines an achromatic diffractive surface with an echelette design. EDOF IOLs have been compared to their aspheric monofocal counterpart suggesting binocular uncorrected intermediate visual acuity (UIVA) and UCNVA of 0.20 or better (Snellen's 20/30) were observed in all cases in the EDOF group, with no significant differences among groups when comparing contrast sensitivity ($p \geq 0.156$) or ocular optical quality parameters ($p \geq 0.084$).[17]

Of the largest studies, Cochener et al, patients were implanted with bilateral EDOF, where one group received nonmonovision set for emmetropia and the other group had a micromonovision (nondominant eye goal –0.50 or –0.75 diopters). Micromonovision increased UIVA and UCNVA. An excellent side effect profile was reported with more than 90% of patients reporting no or mild halos, glare, starbursts, or other photopic phenomena.[18] EDOF IOLs are a great fit for patients who primarily utilize intermediate vision. EDOF IOLs are becoming more and more popular and also have a toric option, which is attractive to many patients and surgeons.

11.3.1 An Ounce of Prevention Is Worth More Than a Pound of Cure

Ideally, careful preoperative assessment and management will mitigate postoperative surprises and other sources for dissatisfaction, and the evaluation and treatment thereof are quite similar pre- and postoperatively. There is no perfect optical system with current presbyopia-correcting IOL designs, and adding ocular disease that affects best-corrected visual acuity (BCVA) may exponentially add to patient dissatisfaction. Thus, a thorough evaluation begins with patient history regarding specific details of timing of when issues began, accurate diagnostics, and optimizing ocular surface, followed by a careful biomicroscopic examination to seek out ocular surface disease (OSD), and corneal and macular pathology. Macular imaging with an optical coherence tomography (OCT) should be performed to identify pathology.

The precorneal tear film must provide a stable tear–corneal interface, and any form of OSD can lead to problems with a rapid tear breakup time (TBUT) and/or punctate epitheliopathy, which will in turn lead to potential sources of refractive surprises and patient dissatisfaction. Along with traditional methods of examining the ocular surface including a TBUT and complete slit-lamp examination (SLE), our assessment of the ocular surface has become much more sophisticated with newer technology testing tear osmolarity and meibography. Epitropoulos and colleagues found significantly greater variability in average keratometric values and anterior corneal astigmatism in those with elevated tear osmolarity, with significant resultant differences in IOL power calculations.[19] These similar clinical diagnostic evaluations apply to before and after cataract surgery. Our treatment and management goes far beyond simple artificial tears, though this first step is at times enough to improve dissatisfaction. Punctal occlusions with temporary or more permanent options are available.[20] Lid hygiene with warm compresses and lid scrubs along with omega fatty acid supplements is an effective start to treating meibomian gland disorder (MGD). Thermal pulsation therapy can have an extended therapeutic effect, lasting upward of 12 months, and can be more effective than the traditional warm compress therapy twice daily.[21] Oral doxycycline or topical azithromycin can be helpful adjunctive therapy for MGD. Other dry eye options include cyclosporine 0.05%, approved to increase tear production, and lifitegrast 5%, which treats signs and symptoms of dry eye disease.[22,23]

Diagnostic imaging modalities provide essential information for the cataract evaluation, but they can also help to identify ocular pathology. Placido disc topography is classically used to determine corneal astigmatism and power, but the placido disc image can provide invaluable insight into the ocular surface. Specifically, irregular and washed-out mires are commonly indicative of dry eye disease or other corneal pathology that contributes to poor image quality. Images with such irregularities can lead to misidentification of corneal power, magnitude, and meridian of the astigmatism. Also, evaluation of the optic nerve or macular disease with a complete dilated examination and OCT imaging is particularly critical to rule out in patients seeking out advanced-technology IOL (ATIOLs), as limited visual potential and decreased contrast sensitivity can lead to a suboptimal quality of vision postoperatively.

Patient expectations are among the most difficult factors to predict, address, and manage when selecting an MFIOL. Understanding patient needs is critical in selecting the appropriate MFIOL. In our modern world of daily computer usage for work, social life, and hobbies, the need for improved intermediate distance is in high demand. When selecting the correct MFIOL, determining the value of the "close vision" needs between intermediate versus near vision for each patient is very important. Other patient-specific considerations include their specific near vision activities, for example, reading with digital reader versus newspaper, and the patient's height that affects the arm span for reading.

11.3.2 Addressing the Less-Than-Satisfied Postoperative Patient

Dissatisfaction after cataract surgery can stem for a myriad of reasons. A systemic and thorough workup is necessary before and after implantation of any ATIOL. Reasons for dissatisfaction include, but are not limited to, anterior chamber (AC) inflammation, macular pathology such as age-related macular degeneration (ARMD) or cystoid macular edema (CME), OSD, residual refractive error, IOL-related issues such as poor quality of vision or dysphotopsia, and IOL malposition. Biomicroscopic examination will identify OSD, inflammation, IOL centration, and/or the position of a toric IOL if such technology was used. The three most cited problems that lead to patient dissatisfaction with MFIOLs are posterior capsular opacification (PCO), OSD, and residual refractive error.[17] Quality-of-vision concerns can also be problematic, including the night vision positive dysphotopsias, dimness to vision with the need for more light with reading, or a diminished quality of central vision or as some call it a "waxy vision."

OSD should be evaluated for and treated thoroughly before consideration of any surgical intervention. Woodward et al demonstrated up to 15% of patient dissatisfaction due to dry eye. Corneal pathology due to dry eye disease, anterior basement membrane dystrophy (ABMD), pterygium, and Salzmann's nodular degeneration (SND) can all lead to inaccurate diagnostics and, thus, a refractive surprise. OSD treatment should proceed as described earlier. In addition, it is necessary to treat OSD exacerbations with preservative-free options, such as dexamethasone (compounded in the United States) or Loteprednol Etabonate ointment. Topical nonsteroidal anti-inflammatory drugs (NSAIDs) can also worsen punctate keratitis, and more modern topical NSAIDs with less-frequent dosing can help mitigate the dry eye disease while still providing the necessary anti-inflammatory benefits. Certain corneal pathology must be surgically managed, including a superficial keratectomy for ABMD and SND or pterygium excisional repair for pterygium.

Woodward et al sited PCO being the most common source of patient dissatisfaction, approaching 60%.[20] Addressing PCO requires a diligent and complete timeline of visual performance, starting from day 1 post-op, week 1 to month 3. If a patient was not satisfied with the quality of their vision in the early post-operative phase, one must critically assess the value added by performing a capsulotomy, especially in MFIOLs, as this can make a refractive exchange much more difficult in the future. After a has patient has healed from surgery and other factors that limit visual acuity have been ruled out, namely, OSD and PCO, residual refractive error should be identified and managed. Post-op ametropia occur due to inaccuracies in the pre-op biometric analysis or limitations of the current calculation formulas available, thus leading to inadequate selection of the IOL power and/or the toricity power. Once a refractive component has been identified as the source of the error, correction options include laser vision correction (LVC), piggyback IOLs, and IOL exchange. Several studies have shown an excellent success rate using laser correction.[24,25] An IOL exchange can be pursued. Kamiya et al reviewed 50 cases of IOL exchange, and demonstrated excellent results, suggesting IOL exchange as an option for the dissatisfied patient. This study reported the most common reason for explanation to be decreased contrast sensitivity (18 eyes, 36%), followed by photic phenomena (17 eyes, 34%).[26]

Another surgical option to correct for pseudophakic residual refractive error is implanting a piggyback IOL. The most serious vision-threatening complication of piggyback IOLs is opacification between the optics of the two lenses, known as interlenticular opacification. The exact mechanism is unclear, but occurs when two IOLs are implanted in the bag. Of importance, such interlenticular opacification has not been reported between an IOL positioned in the sulcus and the second IOL seated within the capsular bag. Options for piggyback IOLs are limited, particularly in the United States. IOLs that have minus power to low plus power

options to correct for low myopic and hyperopic corrections include the J&J Vision Sensar AR40 M (range –10.0 to 1.5 diopters; AR40E 2.0–5.5 diopters), which is a three-piece hydrophobic acrylic monofocal IOL with a 6.0-mm optic diameter, 13.5-mm overall diameter, and a round-edged optic; and the Rayner SulcoFlex (range –7.0 to+7.0), one-piece biocompatible hydrophilic acrylic IOL that comes in toric and multifocal version for sulcus placement, with a 6.5-mm diameter and 14.0-mm overall diameter. The Rayner SulcoFlex is not available in the United States[27] (https://www.humanoptics.com/en/).

As several of the premium IOLs come in toric options, residual astigmatism will provoke patient dissatisfaction. If the residual astigmatism is less than 1.25 diopters, and the patient has a mixed astigmatism, manual corneal relaxing incisions (CRIs) or femtosecond laser arcuate keratotomies (FLAKs) can be an excellent option, particularly if there was an undercorrection of astigmatism and the steep meridian closely coincides with the meridian of the toric IOL. The author has noted that when an overcorrection and a flipped axis have occurred, placement of CRIs or FLAKs in the opposite axis of where the toric IOL is can create a more complicated optical system, and this can compromise the ultimate quality of vision. LVC and toric IOL rotation are also options to tackle residual astigmatic refractive errors. Certain software programs, such as Holladay IOL Consultant Software or one within the iTrace, and the online resource www.astigmatismfix.com, can help surgeons identify if a toric IOL rotation is warranted to neutralize residual astigmatic errors. When facing residual astigmatic errors 1.50 diopters or more, this magnitude of error is beyond the capabilities of arcuate incisions, and toric IOL rotation, IOL exchange, or LVC are the options to work through. When the spherical equivalent is significantly amiss, LVC, piggyback IOLs, and IOL exchange will be options (http://astigmatismfix.com).

One last consideration is the pupil size, high sensitivity for lens centration, and intolerance to kappa angle. The main challenge regarding pupil size is that it is very difficult to predict the pupil size after surgery because it usually changes in comparison with the preoperative measurements. Thus, a very small pupil after the surgery will limit the near vision performance of most of the multifocal lens, while large postoperative pupils are associated with increased photic phenomena. Argon laser iridoplasty has been advocated as the treatment of choice to alleviate IOL decentration, and can also address pupil size with careful planning. Otherwise, a small pupil can be managed with cyclopentolate and a large pupil with brimonidine.[28]

Advanced technology IOLs have expanded the surgeon's armamentarium as to what can be offered to correct distance, intermediate, and near vision during cataract surgery. With all the different options of premium IOLs, surgeons are truly allowed to cater IOL selection to more closely match patients' expectations, needs, and wants. Accommodative lenses have proven to be a good option for patients concerned with visual dysphotopsias, willing to settle with less near vision potential. Bifocal MFIOLs and EDOF have shown to meet the distance, intermediate, and near vision needs. These classes of lenses offer customized options to provide excellent blended vision, with great distance and better intermediate vision, with an improved side effect profile. Surgeons using these lenses will face preoperative and postoperative challenges, but understanding the arsenal available to provide the dissatisfied patient will allow patients to reach their high expectations. In our continued pursuit to provide presbyopia-correcting IOL options for our cataract surgery patients, it is evident we are expanding the effective options that are available to our patients. Understanding the different options available, matched with selecting and explaining the limitations each IOL faces to our patients, will lessen the number of 20/20 vision individuals leaving clinics unhappy, around the world.

11.4 Key Pearls

- The various presbyopia-correcting IOL platforms are discussed including their toric options.
- Preoperative evaluation, including diagnostic technologies, OSD management, and clinical examination, is discussed in detail to help optimize the patient for successful outcomes.
- The importance of setting appropriate expectations and allowing sufficient chair time is discussed.
- Postoperative evaluation and management of the less-than-satisfied patient or the refractive surprise result is discussed.

References

[1] Pepose JS. Maximizing satisfaction with presbyopia-correcting intraocular lenses: the missing links. Am J Ophthalmol. 2008; 146(5):641–648

[2] Heatley CJ, Spalton DJ, Boyce JF, Marshall J. A mathematical model of factors that influence the performance of accommodative intraocular lenses. Ophthalmic Physiol Opt. 2004; 24(2):111–118

[3] Marcos S, Ortiz S, Pérez-Merino P, Birkenfeld J, Durán S, Jiménez-Alfaro I. Three-dimensional evaluation of accommodating intraocular lens shift and alignment in vivo. Ophthalmology. 2014; 121(1):45–55

[4] Stachs O, Schneider H, Beck R, Guthoff R. Pharmacological-induced haptic changes and the accommodative performance in patients with the AT-45 accommodative IOL. J Refract Surg. 2006; 22(2):145–150

[5] Ong HS1. Evans JR, Allan BD. Accommodative intraocular lens versus standard monofocal intraocular lens implantation in cataract surgery. Cochrane Database Syst Rev. 2014; 1:CD009667

[6] Takakura A, Iyer P, Adams JR, Pepin SM. Functional assessment of accommodating intraocular lenses versus monofocal intraocular lenses in cataract surgery: metaanalysis. J Cataract Refract Surg. 2010; 36(3):380–388

[7] Page TP, Whitman J. A stepwise approach for the management of capsular contraction syndrome in hinge-based accommodative intraocular lenses. Clin Ophthalmol. 2016; 10:1039–1046

[8] Forte R, Ursoleo P. The ReZoom multifocal intraocular lens: 2-year follow-up. Eur J Ophthalmol. 2009; 19(3):380–383

[9] Kretz FT, Gerl M, Gerl R, Müller M, Auffarth GU, ZKB00 Study Group. Clinical evaluation of a new pupil independent diffractive multifocal intraocular lens with a + 2.75 D near addition: a European multicentre study. Br J Ophthalmol. 2015; 99(12):1655–1659

[10] Kretz FT, Koss MJ, Auffarth GU, ZLB00 Study Group. Intermediate and near visual acuity of an aspheric, bifocal, diffractive multifocal intraocular lens with + 3.25 D near addition. J Refract Surg. 2015; 31(5):295–299

[11] Lubiński W, Gronkowska-Serafin J, Podborączyńska-Jodko K. Clinical outcomes after cataract surgery with implantation of the Tecnis ZMB00 multifocal intraocular lens. Med Sci Monit. 2014; 20:1220–1226

[12] Mastropasqua R, Pedrotti E, Passilongo M, Parisi G, Marchesoni I, Marchini G. Long-term visual function and patient satisfaction after bilateral implantation and combination of two similar multifocal IOLs. J Refract Surg. 2015; 31(5):308–314

[13] Kim JS, Jung JW, Lee JM, Seo KY, Kim EK, Kim TI. Clinical outcomes following implantation of diffractive multifocal intraocular lenses with varying add powers. Am J Ophthalmol. 2015; 160(4):702–9.e1

[14] Gibbons A, Ali TK, Waren DP, Donaldson KE. Causes and correction of dissatisfaction after implantation of presbyopia-correcting intraocular lenses. Clin Ophthalmol. 2016; 10: 1965–1970

[15] Vega F, Millán MS, Vila-Terricabras N, Alba-Bueno F. Visible versus near-infrared optical performance of diffractive multifocal intraocular lenses. Invest Ophthalmol Vis Sci. 2015; 56 (12):7345–7351

[16] Carson D, Hill WE, Hong X, Karakelle M. Optical bench performance of AcrySof(®) IQ ReSTOR(®), AT LISA(®) tri, and FineVision(®) intraocular lenses. Clin Ophthalmol. 2014; 8: 2105–2113

[17] Pedrotti E, Bruni E, Bonacci E, Badalamenti R, Mastropasqua R, Marchini G. Comparative analysis of the clinical outcomes with a monofocal and an extended range of vision intraocular lens. J Refract Surg. 2016; 32(7):436–442

[18] Cochener B, Concerto Study Group. Clinical outcomes of a new extended range of vision intraocular lens: international multicenter concerto study. J Cataract Refract Surg. 2016; 42 (9):1268–1275

[19] Epitropoulos AT, Matossian C, Berdy GJ, Malhotra RP, Potvin R. Effect of tear osmolarity on repeatability of keratometry for cataract surgery planning. J Cataract Refract Surg. 2015; 41(8):1672–1677

[20] Woodward MA, Randleman JB, Stulting RD. Dissatisfaction after multifocal intraocular lens implantation. J Cataract Refract Surg. 2009; 35(6):992–997

[21] Blackie CA, Coleman CA, Holland EJ. The sustained effect (12 months) of a single-dose vectored thermal pulsation procedure for meibomian gland dysfunction and evaporative dry eye. Clin Ophthalmol. 2016; 10:1385–1396

[22] Allergan, Inc. Restasis [package insert]. Irvine, CA: Allergan, Inc; 2013

[23] Sheppard JD, Torkildsen GL, Lonsdale JD, et al. OPUS-1 Study Group. Lifitegrast ophthalmic solution 5.0% for treatment of dry eye disease: results of the OPUS-1 phase 3 study. Ophthalmology. 2014; 121(2):475–483

[24] Piñero DR, Ayala Espinosa MJ, Alió JL. LASIK outcomes following multifocal and monofocal intraocular lens implantation. J Refract Surg. 2010; 26(8):569–577

[25] Muftuoglu O, Prasher P, Chu C, et al. Laser in situ keratomileusis for residual refractive errors after apodized diffractive multifocal intraocular lens implantation. J Cataract Refract Surg. 2009; 35(6):1063–1071

[26] Kamiya K, Hayashi K, Shimizu K, Negishi K, Sato M, Bissen-Miyajima H, Survey Working Group of the Japanese Society of Cataract and Refractive Surgery. Multifocal intraocular lens explantation: a case series of 50 eyes. Am J Ophthalmol. 2014; 158(2):215–220.e1

[27] Manzouri B, Dari M, Claoué C. Supplementary IOLs: monofocal and multifocal, their applications and limitations. Asia Pac J Ophthalmol (Phila). 2017; 6(4):358–363

[28] Alio JL, Plaza-Puche AB, Férnandez-Buenaga R, Pikkel J, Maldonado M. Multifocal intraocular lenses: an overview. Surv Ophthalmol. 2017; 62(5):611–634

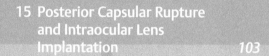

Part III

**Nonrefractive Enhancement
Procedures**

12 Dysphotopsias and Surgical Management

Samuel Masket and Nicole R. Fram

Abstract

As dysphotopsia is a subjective phenomenon, it is difficult to predict as to which patients will experience dysphotopsia following an uneventful surgery. Some patients may be particularly vulnerable or particularly sensitive to dysphotopsia and may require additional surgical treatment. Reverse optic capture, piggyback intraocular lens (IOL) implantation, and sulcus placement of an IOL are considered surgical mode for nonabating negative dysphotopsia. Positive dysphotopsias (PDs) are often associated with thick optic-edge IOLs and IOLs with high index of refraction. PD patients who do not respond to medical line of therapy often need an IOL exchange.

Keywords: dysphotopsia, negative dysphotopsia, positive dysphotopsia, reverse optic capture, secondary reverse optic capture, photophobia, glare

12.1 Introduction

Negative dysphotopsia (ND) represents an undesired optical phenomenon following cataract surgery. It is classically described as a dark temporal shadow. Conversely, positive dysphotopsia (PD) is characterized by light streaks, starbursts, or glare. Both photopsias interfere significantly with the quality of vision and perceived success of surgery. The dysphotopsias can result in unrelenting patient dissatisfaction after otherwise uncomplicated cataract surgery. Given that ND and PD differ in etiology and management, techniques for treatment should be considered separately. However, both conditions may exist simultaneously.

12.2 Negative Dysphotopsia

ND, first described by Davison as a dark shadow in the temporal visual field, is an undesired optical phenomenon that may follow otherwise uncomplicated contemporary cataract surgery in which an intraocular lens (IOL) is placed in the capsule bag remnant with an overlying continuous circular anterior capsulotomy.[1,2] As noted in the present report and by others, ND has been reported with a variety of IOLs[2,3] and ND was not described prior to capsulorrhexis and has not been associated with malpositioned IOLs. Although the etiology remains uncertain and is likely multifactorial, several mechanisms have been proposed. Holladay et al, in their original report using ray tracing in a nonclinical study, implicated square-edge design IOLs, increased posterior chamber depth, small pupil diameter, and high index of refraction IOLs among other factors as causal of ND.[4] In a more recent study, Holladay et al, again employing ray-tracing nonclinical studies, revised their original theory to include nasal anterior capsule overlap, IOL optic shape, high IOL power, high angle kappa (chord mu), small pupil, optic asphericity, etc., as theoretically causes of ND; they no longer limit IOL optic-edge character and iris–optic distance as primary factors.[5] Interestingly, their recent observations are more consistent with our original clinical findings that implicate the overlapped anterior nasal capsule.[2,5]

Diagnostic tests to rule out concomitant ocular pathology including visual field testing and a thorough dilated fundus retinal examination are needed prior to attributing symptoms to persistent ND. Unfortunately, medical treatment has not been shown to be useful in treating ND. Initial reports implicated temporal corneal incisions as a causative factor in ND[6]; however, ND has been reported with superior incisions.[7] Previous publications have implicated posterior chamber depth, pupil size, index of refraction, lens material, and edge design as causative factors in ND.[4] Vámosi et al concluded that in-the-bag IOL exchange alone did not improve symptoms of ND and posterior chamber depth as examined by ultrasound biomicroscopy (UBM) was not a significant factor in incidence of ND.[8] However, with sulcus placement of the IOL during exchange, symptoms of ND were improved. Although the etiology of ND is likely multifactorial, we do know that it can occur with any lens material, is persistent despite collapse of the posterior chamber with an "in-the-bag" IOL, and does not typically improve with in-the-bag IOL exchange. This constellation of findings implicates the anterior capsule–IOL interaction as a possible factor in the etiology of ND.[2,4]

Surgical methods to address ND include secondary "piggyback" IOL, reverse optic capture (ROC), and/or sulcus placement of a secondary posterior chamber IOL (PCIOL), which have all been devised and proven useful in reducing visual symptoms of ND. Although ND rarely induces visual disability sufficient to require an operative approach, some patients are very disturbed and can be very vocal in their complaints. To our understanding, ND has never been reported with sulcus placed PCIOLs or anterior chamber IOLs (ACIOLs). In our investigation, we found that ND occurs only with "in-the-bag" PCIOLs with overlap of the anterior capsulorrhexis onto the anterior surface of the PCIOL.[2] We do not believe that the corneal incision plays a role in persistent ND.[6]

Given the above, and in keeping with our studies, two surgical strategies have emerged as beneficial: ROC and placement of a secondary "piggyback" IOL. Failed surgical strategies include bag-to-bag IOL exchange wherein the original implant is removed and another of different material, shape, or edge design is replaced within the capsule bag. This is in keeping with the work of Vámosi et al.[2,8]

One successful surgical method, ROC, may be employed as a secondary surgery for symptomatic patients or as a primary prophylactic strategy. In the case of the latter, the method has been applied to the second eye of patients who were significantly symptomatic following routine uncomplicated surgery in their first eye. It should be noted,

however, that ND symptoms are not necessarily bilateral.

Secondary ROC, performed for symptomatic patients, may be applied if the anterior capsulotomy is not too small or too thick or rigid from postoperative fibrosis. At surgery, the anterior capsule is freed from the underlying optic by gentle blunt and viscodissection (▸ Fig. 12.1). Next, the nasal anterior capsule edge is retracted with one Sinskey hook (or similar device), while the optic edge is elevated and the capsule edge allowed to slip under the optic (▸ Fig. 12.2). This maneuver is

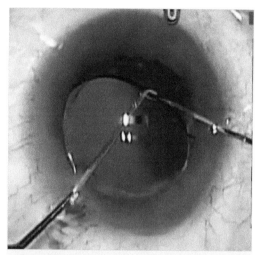

Fig. 12.2 The Sinskey hook and blunt spatula are used to elevate the optic edge over the capsule.

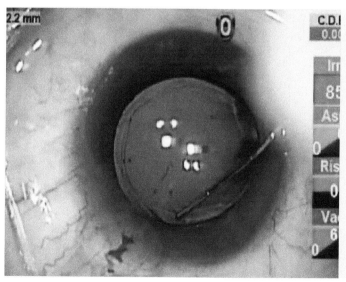

Fig. 12.1 A Sinskey hook is fed underneath the anterior capsule following viscodissection in an attempt to free the optic from the capsule.

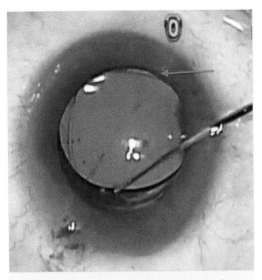

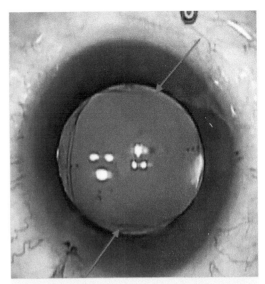

Fig. 12.3 Once the nasal edge has been captured (*arrow*), the opposite, temporal edge of the optic is elevated over the anterior capsule edge.

Fig. 12.4 Optic capture has been completed. The nasal and temporal edges of the implant are anterior to the anterior capsule (*arrows*), whereas the haptics remain fully within the capsular bag.

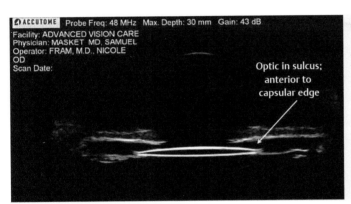

Optic in sulcus; anterior to capsular edge

Fig. 12.5 Ultrasound biomicroscopy (UBM) demonstrating reverse optic capture with the optic-edge anterior to the capsular edge.

repeated 180 degrees away temporally, leaving the haptics undisturbed in the bag (▶ Fig. 12.3, ▶ Fig. 12.4, ▶ Fig. 12.5, ▶ Fig. 12.6). Primary or prophylactic ROC is performed at the time of initial cataract surgery for the symptomatic patient's second eye. It should be recognized that surgical success in achieving primary or secondary ROC is highly dependent on a properly sized and centered anterior capsulorhexis. There seems to be little optical consequence of ROC, as the haptics remain in the bag; theoretically, however, a modest myopic shift would be induced, varying directly with the power of the IOL. There have been no reported cases of iris chafing with ROC; however,

we have had cases of iris chafing associated with piggyback PCIOLs.

The other surgical method that has proven successful for patients with symptomatic ND is a "piggyback" IOL, as first reported by Ernest.[9] In this method, a second IOL is implanted in the ciliary sulcus atop the IOL–capsule bag complex. It appears that covering the primary optic–capsule junction reduces ND symptoms, although the original concept was that a "piggyback" lens was effective because it collapsed the posterior chamber by reducing the distance between the posterior iris and the anterior surface of the IOL. However, our studies have determined that the depth of the

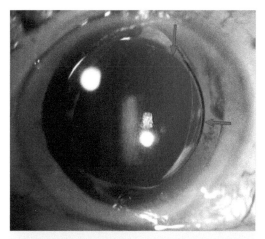

Fig. 12.6 Slit-lamp photo of secondary reverse optic capture (SROC). Note that the optic overlays the nasal anterior capsule (*arrows*).

posterior chamber is unrelated to ND symptoms.[8] We prefer use of a three-piece silicone or collamer IOL. Regarding ametropia and piggyback IOLs, for hyperopic errors multiply the spectacle error by 1.5 to determine IOL power, while for myopic errors multiply by 1.2. So, as an example, in the case of a 2-diopter hyperope, implant a + 3.0 diopter IOL in the ciliary sulcus.

Recent publications have reported improvement of ND symptoms with neodymium:yttrium aluminum garnet (Nd:YAG) capsulectomy of the nasal anterior capsule.[10,11] This treatment, however, may limit future management strategies such as ROC in the event that the capsulectomy intervention is unsuccessful. Further, there is no current standardization of how much nasal capsule should be removed to alleviate the symptoms.

Finally, Henderson et al also suggested that ND occurrence with single-piece acrylic IOLs may be reduced in the early postoperative period if the haptics are oriented horizontally rather than vertically.[12] The idea of a potentially preventative strategy is encouraging. However, they noted in their study that the preventative benefit was not statistically significant between the horizontally and vertically oriented IOL haptics after 1 month.[12] Although we have not investigated their strategy, we continue to observe ND with horizontal orientation of single-piece acrylic IOLs. This is not surprising as our investigation concerns patients with long-standing ND. Additionally, Mahar reported three of three patients with ND who had single-piece acrylic IOLs with horizontal orientation of

the haptics.[13] Therefore, it appears that specific haptic orientation may not prove to be a meaningful long-term strategy for treatment of persistent ND, though it might be beneficial to reduce early incidence.

12.3 Positive Dysphotopsia

PD is reported by patients as light streaks, halos, starbursts, etc. It may be induced by internal reflections from either the optic edge or optic surfaces.[14,15,16,17,18] Therefore, PD appears to be related directly to IOL material, optic size index of refraction, radius of curvature, surface reflectivity, and edge design. Typically, PD is associated with thick square-edge design, high index of refraction, low radius of curvature, and high surface reflectivity.[15,16,17,18] Unlike ND, patients may perceive benefit from use of miotic agents, particularly under dim-light conditions. Medical management of PD includes brimonidine tartrate 0.15% initially; also useful is a dilute solution of pilocarpine, typically 0.5%. While topical miotics may be helpful, they are associated with the potential for allergies and side effects.

Should miotic therapy prove unsuccessful, and the symptoms mandate further treatment, IOL exchange may be highly successful. In this situation, opt for a lens with a low index of refraction, large optic diameter, and a thin round-edge design. Unfortunately, there are no fully round-edge IOLs currently available in the United States. Therefore, the only surgical option for potential resolution is to change the IOL material.

ND must be distinguished from PD in that the latter is characterized by patient complaints of peripheral light arcs, halos, or central light flashes. PD may coexist with ND and there can be symptom crossover between the two conditions.[1] The etiology of PD has been more clearly established than that of ND; most agree that PD is induced by internal light reflection by the truncated square edge of IOLs and by the flat radius of curvature of the anterior surface of high index of refraction IOLs.[17,18] When ND and PD coexist, corrective surgery must address both conditions. The IOL material change is to address the PD and the ROC or sulcus position is to address the ND.

Patients with either ND or PD require careful and concerned attention to their symptoms, a meaningful discussion of the suspected etiology, and should be presented with a supportive plan for assistance.

12.4 Key Pearls

- It is essential to differentiate between ND and PD as the former is marked by the presence of dark temporal crescent, whereas the latter is marked by positive streaks, glare, and photophobia.
- The complaints of dysphotopsia are marked in the initial postoperative period and they often wane off after few months. Only dysphotopsias that are persistent over a longer duration of time should be considered for surgical intervention.
- Secondary ROC, piggyback IOLs, and sulcus placement of the IOLs are often helpful in overcoming the symptoms of ND.
- PD often requires an IOL exchange if unresponsive to medical line of treatment with miotics.

References

[1] Davison JA. Positive and negative dysphotopsia in patients with acrylic intraocular lenses. J Cataract Refract Surg. 2000; 26(9):1346–1355

[2] Masket S, Fram NR. Pseudophakic negative dysphotopsia: Surgical management and new theory of etiology. J Cataract Refract Surg. 2011; 37(7):1199–1207

[3] Trattler WB, Whitsett JC, Simone PA. Negative dysphotopsia after intraocular lens implantation irrespective of design and material. J Cataract Refract Surg. 2005; 31(4):841–845

[4] Holladay JT, Zhao H, Reisin CR. Negative dysphotopsia: the enigmatic penumbra. J Cataract Refract Surg. 2012; 38(7):1251–1265

[5] Holladay JT, Simpson MJ. Negative dysphotopsia: Causes and rationale for prevention and treatment. J Cataract Refract Surg. 2017; 43(2):263–275

[6] Osher RH. Negative dysphotopsia: long-term study and possible explanation for transient symptoms. J Cataract Refract Surg. 2008; 34(10):1699–1707

[7] Cooke DL. Negative dysphotopsia after temporal corneal incisions. J Cataract Refract Surg. 2010; 36(4):671–672

[8] Vámosi P, Csákány B, Németh J. Intraocular lens exchange in patients with negative dysphotopsia symptoms. J Cataract Refract Surg. 2010; 36(3):418–424

[9] Ernest PH. Severe photic phenomenon. J Cataract Refract Surg. 2006; 32(4):685–686

[10] Cooke DL, Kasko S, Platt LO. Resolution of negative dysphotopsia after laser anterior capsulotomy. J Cataract Refract Surg. 2013; 39(7):1107–1109

[11] Folden DV. Neodymium:YAG laser anterior capsulectomy: surgical option in the management of negative dysphotopsia. J Cataract Refract Surg. 2013; 39(7):1110–1115

[12] Henderson BA, Yi DH, Constantine JB, Geneva II. New preventative approach for negative dysphotopsia. J Cataract Refract Surg. 2016; 42(10):1449–1455

[13] Mahar PS. Negative Dysphotopsia after Uncomplicated Phacoemulsification. Pak J Ophthalmol.. 2013; 29(1):53–56

[14] Holladay JT, Lang A, Portney V. Analysis of edge glare phenomena in intraocular lens edge designs. J Cataract Refract Surg. 1999; 25(6):748–752

[15] Masket S. Truncated edge design, dysphotopsia, and inhibition of posterior capsule opacification. J Cataract Refract Surg. 2000; 26(1):145–147

[16] Masket S, Geraghty E, Crandall AS, et al. Undesired light images associated with ovoid intraocular lenses. J Cataract Refract Surg. 1993; 19(6):690–694

[17] Franchini A, Gallarati BZ, Vaccari E. Computerized analysis of the effects of intraocular lens edge design on the quality of vision in pseudophakic patients. J Cataract Refract Surg. 2003; 29(2):342–347

[18] Erie JC, Bandhauer MH, McLaren JW. Analysis of postoperative glare and intraocular lens design. J Cataract Refract Surg. 2001; 27(4):614–621

13 Bullous Keratopathy and Endothelial Keratoplasty

Jonathan K. Kam and Jacqueline Beltz

Abstract

Persistent corneal stromal edema with associated epithelial bullae following intraocular surgery is termed corneal decompensation or bullous keratopathy. This may account for a suboptimal outcome following cataract surgery. Identifying a patient at risk of corneal decompensation allows for appropriate counseling in relation to the increased risk of an adverse outcome, and management options should that adverse outcome occur. This chapter describes the clinical features of bullous keratopathy and how to identify a patient at risk of developing bullous keratopathy. Surgical considerations such as preoperative workup, intraocular lens selection, and appropriate modifications to cataract surgery for these patients will be discussed. The chapter will also address the diagnosis and management of bullous keratopathy.

Keywords: bullous keratopathy, corneal edema, endothelial cell loss, endothelial dystrophy, endothelial keratoplasty, Descemet's stripping automated endothelial keratoplasty, Descemet's membrane endothelial keratoplasty

13.1 Introduction

Persistent corneal stromal edema following intraocular surgery with associated epithelial bullae is termed bullous keratopathy. The term aphakic or pseudophakic is added, depending on the lens status of the eye (ABK/PBK). These conditions are characterized by endothelial cell compromise causing pain and loss of vision. ABK and PBK are important causes of poor visual outcomes following cataract surgery, and are a leading indication for keratoplasty.[1]

Frequent causes of corneal endothelial failure include prior intraocular surgery, corneal endothelial dystrophy, or failure of an existing corneal transplant. Other less common causes include trauma, acute-angle closure glaucoma, and iridocorneal endothelial syndrome. Certain conditions, such as prior ocular trauma, prolonged or complicated cataract surgery, retained crystalline lens fragments, toxic anterior segment syndrome (TASS), unstable intraocular lenses (IOLs), or glaucoma drainage devices, may increase the risk of significant endothelial cell loss, although all intraocular surgery would be expected to cause some cell loss.

Bullous keratopathy may account for a suboptimal outcome following cataract surgery in patients with or without risk factors. If a patient does have risk factors, preoperative counseling and surgical planning are essential in achieving the best possible outcome for the patient. If bullous keratopathy does occur, a good outcome with a satisfied patient will depend on good communication and appropriate management. Patients with preexisting corneal endothelial cell failure might benefit from a combined procedure, most commonly cataract surgery combined with endothelial keratoplasty (EK). If cataract surgery is planned alone, intraocular surgery may be modified to reduce the chance of further endothelial cell loss. If endothelial cell failure does occur and persist, then EK might be considered as a secondary procedure. Identifying risk factors, performing preoperative workup, modifying cataract surgery, selecting an appropriate IOL, and diagnosing and managing postcataract surgery bullous keratopathy will be the focus of this chapter.

13.2 Risk Factor Identification

Careful examination of the cornea is an important part of the preoperative workup for cataract surgery. Identifying a patient at risk allows for appropriate counseling in relation to the increased risk of the procedure, potential for adverse outcome, and management options should that adverse outcome occur.

Preoperative Considerations

- Corneal guttata.
- Pseudoexfoliation (PXF).
- Angle-closure glaucoma.
- Density of cataract.
- Corneal endothelial dystrophy:
  - Fuchs' endothelial corneal dystrophy.
  - Congenital hereditary endothelial dystrophy.
  - Posterior polymorphous dystrophy.
  - X-linked corneal endothelial dystrophy.
- Postinfectious:
  - Herpes simplex virus.
  - Herpes zoster virus.

○ Cytomegalovirus.
- Postintraocular surgery:
  ○ Number, type, and complexity of previous intraocular procedures.
- Past ocular trauma.
- Iridocorneal endothelial syndrome.

The most important factors to identify preoperatively are the presence of corneal guttata and/or abnormalities in endothelial cell count or morphology. A history of prior intraocular surgery, acute-angle closure glaucoma, ocular trauma, or previous significant corneal infections might suggest increased risk, prompting further investigation. Preoperative slit-lamp examination would routinely be used to assess type and density of cataract, and any specific challenging features. Risk factors for corneal edema should be considered at the same time.

Corneal guttae are small excrescences on Descemet's membrane (DM) that occur due to overproduction of basement membrane (▶ Fig. 13.1). They may occur peripherally as part of normal aging, but are considered pathologic and are associated with Fuchs' endothelial corneal dystrophy (FECD) when they occur centrally. In FECD, corneal guttae are often associated with progressive endothelial cell loss and corneal edema[2] and this may be further exacerbated by intraocular surgery.

Corneal guttae are best identified at the slit lamp on retroillumination with a dilated pupil (▶ Fig. 13.2). Appearance is of a dimpled endothelium sometimes described as a beaten metal appearance. Guttata may be sporadic, diffuse, or confluent. Confluent guttae are more likely to be visually symptomatic than sporadic corneal guttata. Corneal edema is visible by either folds in DM, generalized haze, microcystic change, or opacity.

Pseudoexfoliation (PXF) syndrome is an important risk factor to identify due to the increased risk of surgical complication, as well as an association with abnormal DM and increased rate of endothelial cell loss.[3] Early identification of these risk factors allows for counseling of the patient prior to cataract surgery, consideration of appropriate surgical modifications, selection of an appropriate IOL, and/or consideration of cataract surgery combined with corneal transplant procedure.

The surgeon and patient should discuss the severity and impact of both the cataract and the corneal endothelial disease. Symptoms such as early morning blur that clears throughout the day

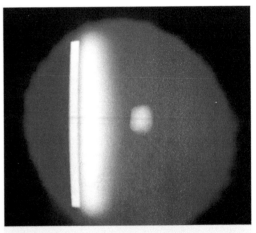

Fig. 13.2 Corneal guttata as appreciated on retroillumination on slit lamp.

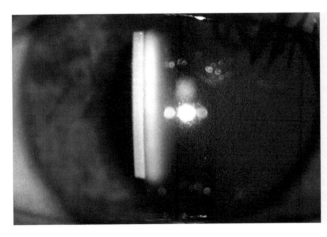

Fig. 13.1 Slit-lamp photo demonstrating corneal guttata.

and difficulty driving at night may indicate symptomatic endothelial cell disease. The visual requirements of the patient and clinical features of both their cataract and corneal disease will help determine the most appropriate procedure, whether that be cataract surgery alone or cataract surgery combined with EK.

13.3 Preoperative Workup

Once a patient has been identified as at increased risk for corneal endothelial cell failure, further preoperative investigation is warranted. Central corneal thickness should be measured and documented. Specular microscopy may be beneficial,

not only to quantify risk, but also to aid in patient counseling. Endothelial cell density and morphology can be considered (▶ Fig. 13.3, ▶ Fig. 13.4, ▶ Fig. 13.5).

Accuracy of biometry is often reduced in the setting of endothelial disease. This may lead to difficulty in IOL selection. Biometry should be performed as early as possible on patients with potential for corneal decompensation, ideally prior to progression of their corneal disease. It may also be useful to compare the biometry to the other eye, which may have a more normal endothelial appearance. Keratometry values are difficult to quantify, and particularly axis of astigmatism can be difficult in the presence of endothelial disease.

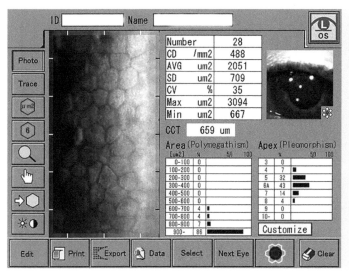

Fig. 13.3 Specular microscopy in a patient with a low endothelial cell count and a high degree of polymegathism and pleomorphism.

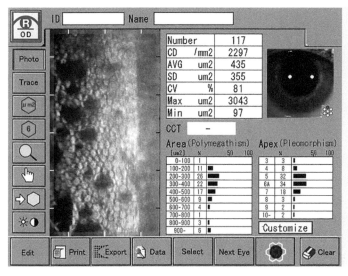

Fig. 13.4 Specular microscopy showing midperipheral corneal guttata with healthy intervening corneal endothelial cells.

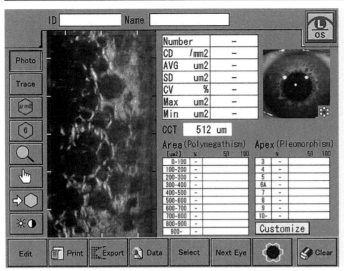

Fig. 13.5 Specular microscopy showing more advanced central corneal guttata with minimal intervening endothelial cells.

Measuring keratometry values by multiple methods is recommended. The various factors that influence the decision to perform a cataract surgery alone versus the combined procedure are highlighted.

Preoperative Investigations

- Central corneal thickness.
- Specular microscopy.
- Biometry.
- Corneal tomography/topography.
- Manual keratometry.

Factors Influencing Decision to do Cataract Surgery Alone versus Combined Procedure

- Severity and impact of each feature.
- Symptoms (early morning blur).
- Visual requirements of patient.
- Degree/confluence of guttata.
- Increasing/asymmetric corneal thickness.
- Epithelial or stromal edema.

13.4 Intraocular Lens Selection

IOL selection is complex in the presence of corneal endothelial disease, due to a difficulty in gaining accurate preoperative measurements, as well as the uncertain effect on corneal function and therefore power postoperatively. In addition, if the patient goes on to require EK, the corneal power will further change, and that change will be unpredictable.

General considerations include the type of IOL, the material of the IOL, and the power. Monofocal IOLs are usually appropriate. Multifocal IOLs and extended depth of focus IOLs are generally not recommended for patients with endothelial cell compromise. Toric IOLs may have a place, and should be considered on a case-by-case basis depending on accuracy and reproducibility of measurements. Hydrophilic material is known to have the potential to opacify when it comes into contact with air or gas. There have been several cases reported of IOL opacity post-EK in patients with hydrophilic IOLs.[4] It is therefore recommended to avoid hydrophilic IOLs in patients who may go on to require EK in the future.

EK is associated with a hyperopic shift, of varying magnitude. The reason for this is multifactorial, and includes the addition of a concave lenticule (in the case of DSAEK), and an unpredictable amount of corneal deturgescence with Descemet's stripping automated endothelial keratoplasty (DSAEK) and DM endothelial keratoplasty (DMEK). Up to 1.5-diopter hyperopic shift in spherical equivalent has been reported after DSAEK,[5] and a lesser shift after ultrathin (UT) DSAEK[6] and DMEK.[7] The range is great, and predictability is difficult. Common targets for patients undergoing combined cataract surgery and EK would be –0.5 - –0.75 for DMEK and –0.75 - –1.5D for DSAEK or UT DSAEK. If the patient is undergoing cataract surgery alone, this hyperopic shift should still be taken into account, in case EK is required in the future. Surgeons should then aim to reduce the chance of postoperative hypermetropia where possible, by selecting a myopic target.

13.5 Surgical Considerations

Surgery can be adapted to minimize the endothelial cell loss during cataract surgery in patients who are at increased risk.

Endothelial cell loss can be minimized by performing phacoemulsification away from the cornea in the iris plane and minimizing the phacoemulsification energy emitted. For dense cataracts, using a dispersive and cohesive ophthalmic viscoelastic device (OVD) with a soft-shell technique has been shown to lower endothelial cell loss at 3 months, when compared to a cohesive OVD alone.[8,9] Advanced phacoemulsification technologies such as torsional ultrasound likely reduce the energy.[10,11] Nuclear disassembly by phaco-chop as opposed to divide and conquer has been shown to be beneficial in the moderately dense cases.[12] A number of different phacoemulsification handpiece tips have been reported recently, but have not been shown to greatly alter endothelial cell loss.[13] For very dense cataracts, manual small-incision cataract surgery (MSICS) might provide some advantage. However, a meta-analysis of randomized controlled trials found that there were no significant differences in endothelial cell loss between the two techniques. Phacoemulsification was superior to MSICS in uncorrected visual acuity and caused less surgically induced astigmatism.[14,15,16] For all of these, technique adaptations, surgeon skill, and experience should be considered, as the most important factor is the avoidance of surgical complications.

Several features of the irrigating solution may impact the endothelial cell loss. Time, volume, and chemical composition might be considered. No difference in endothelial cell loss at 6 months was found when fortified balanced salt solution (BSS) was compared with Ringer's lactate irrigating solution.[17] Solutions such as BSS Plus (glucose glutathione bicarbonate solution) approximate characteristics of aqueous humor and therefore might provide a theoretical advantage; however, Lucena et al found no significant difference in endothelial cell loss using Ringer's solution when compared to BSS Plus.[18]

Intracameral medications such as anesthetic agents, mydriatic agents, and antibiotic agents are frequently used during cataract surgery. One must ensure that the correct concentration of any drug is used to avoid corneal toxicity. Preservative-free lidocaine from 0.1 to 0.5 mL has been found to show no change in endothelial cell count at 3 months, but higher concentrations can cause significant endothelial cell loss.[19]

Performing femtosecond laser-assisted cataract surgery (FLACS) can reduce the cumulative phacoemulsification energy needed to emulsify and extract a cataract.[20] Whether FLACS causes significantly less endothelial cell loss in the long term compared to conventional cataract surgery is unclear.[21,22,23] In a prospective comparative cohort study, corneal edema was significantly less with FLACS compared to conventional surgery at 1 day and 3 weeks postoperatively. However, the difference was negligible at 6 months. In the same study, FLACS had significantly less endothelial cell loss at 3 weeks but not at 6 months. Interestingly, eyes that had laser-automated corneal incisions had greater endothelial cell loss at 6 months than eyes with manual corneal incisions.[23] A meta-analysis of 9 randomized controlled trials and 15 cohort studies suggested that FLACS is a safer and more effective method for reducing endothelial cell loss than conventional phacoemulsification surgery.[24] It is important to note that this conclusion was based mainly on evidence at 3 months postoperatively and that few studies extended follow-up beyond that time.

Cataract surgery complicated with vitreous loss is associated with increased endothelial cell loss, and an increased rate of corneal edema.[25] Retained nuclear fragments in the anterior chamber can also lead to corneal decompensation.[26] When the capsular support is lost, IOL placement must be considered. In a comparative study of IOL placement following complicated cataract surgery, there was no difference in the incidence of corneal decompensation following primary anterior chamber IOL (ACIOL; 12.4%) and secondary scleral-fixated IOL (10.8%) implantation.[27]

13.5.1 Diagnosis of Bullous Keratopathy

Corneal edema may occur in the early postoperative period after cataract surgery, and in many cases will resolve. Failure to resolve or start improving by 4 weeks postoperatively should start to raise the possibility of persisting bullous keratopathy.

A differential diagnosis should be considered, especially if the findings are unexpected and if the patient did not have preexisting risk factors or

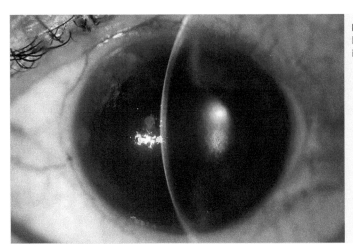

Fig. 13.6 Slit-lamp photo of bullous keratopathy and posterior chamber intraocular lens.

complicated surgery. DM detachment is important to identify, as this is potentially reversible. DM detachment can be identified at the slit lamp by the presence of a double anterior chamber, particularly with a bright and narrow slit-lamp beam. Anterior segment ocular coherence tomography (ASOCT) may show the detachment. Reattachment may be possible with an injection of air. The surgical procedure and other patients on the same operating list might be considered to help rule out endothelial toxicity or toxic anterior segment syndrome (TASS). Raised intraocular pressure might be associated with microcystic corneal edema that may resolve on normalization of the IOP. Endophthalmitis is associated with pain as well as pan ocular inflammation.

> **Differential Diagnosis of Bullous Keratopathy**
>
> - DM detachment.
> - Endothelial toxicity/TASS.
> - Raised IOP.
> - Endophthalmitis.

13.5.2 Clinical Features of Bullous Keratoplasty

Bullous keratopathy can be diagnosed by history, examination, and investigations. Reduced vision is worse on waking, and improving as the day progresses is typical. A patient may have foreign body sensation or pain if open bullae are present. They may also have some photophobia. Examination

findings include corneal thickening, DM folds, and cystic bullae (▶ Fig. 13.6, ▶ Fig. 13.7, ▶ Fig. 13.8). Pachymetry shows an increased corneal thickness, while specular microscopy reveals a decreased endothelial cell density and may demonstrate the presence of guttae, although adequate imaging may not be possible through significant corneal edema. ASOCT can be useful to measure corneal thickness and identify DM flaps.

13.6 Management of Bullous Keratopathy

Initial treatment is most often conservative. Resolution may be unlikely if significant improvement has not been noted by 3 months. Topical antibiotic should be considered for infectious prophylaxis. Topical steroids might help reduce the inflammatory component during the early postoperative period. Topical hypertonic saline (sodium chloride 5%) might help reduce epithelial edema and provide some symptomatic relief. Intraocular pressure should be controlled. Carbonic anhydrase inhibitors should be avoided if possible, as there is a possibility of worsening the edema.[28] A bandage contact lens might be required during this period if discomfort is significant. If conservative measures fail, EK is the treatment of choice for corneal endothelial failure in eyes that have visual potential. If visual potential is poor, alternative surgical options such as phototherapeutic keratectomy (PTK) or Gunderson's flap could be considered. If a retained nuclear fragment or unstable IOL is causing progressive inflammation and endothelial cell loss, then removal of the offending entity is recommended.

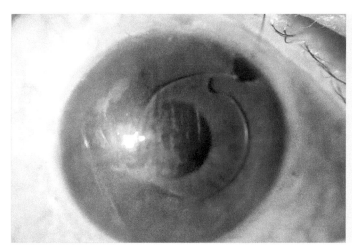

Fig. 13.7 Slit-lamp photo of corneal endothelial failure and poorly positioned anterior chamber intraocular lens.

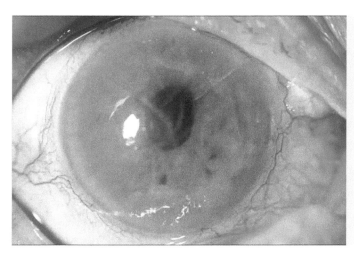

Fig. 13.8 Slit-lamp photo of corneal endothelial failure and a long and anteriorly placed glaucoma drainage device.

13.7 Endothelial Keratoplasty

If corneal edema persists at 4 weeks postoperatively, referral to a corneal specialist is appropriate. While intervention may be best delayed until 3 months after cataract surgery, the patient may benefit from early referral. Preoperative explanation and counseling can commence, and a surgical date can be arranged if necessary.

DSAEK is now established as the gold standard for the surgical management of bullous keratopathy. This is due to the reduced intraoperative risk, improved visual outcomes, reduced rejection rates, and faster visual recovery when compared to penetrating keratoplasty (▶ Fig. 13.9, ▶ Fig. 13.10, ▶ Fig. 13.11, ▶ Fig. 13.12).[29] In 2006, Melles introduced DMEK[30] with the aim of further improving visual outcomes. In comparison with DSAEK, DMEK has shown faster visual recovery,[31,32]

improved visual outcomes,[31,32,33] and reduced rejection rates.[31,34,35] DMEK, however, remains less popular than DSAEK, due to the increased technically difficulty and the increased intraoperative and postoperative risks.[36]

In 2011, it was suggested that DSAEK utilizing thinner donor tissue achieved better visual acuity than those with thicker donor tissue.[37] In order to test the hypothesis that thin tissue was associated with improved visual outcomes, Busin developed a technique to prospectively produce thin tissue, which he termed UT-DSAEK.[6] It has since become apparent that thickness alone may not be responsible for the improved visual outcomes, but that irregularities in stromal shape and thickness may be important and that these irregularities might be less likely when the stromal component of the graft is less.[38] Several techniques are now used by surgeons and eye banks to reproducibly obtain

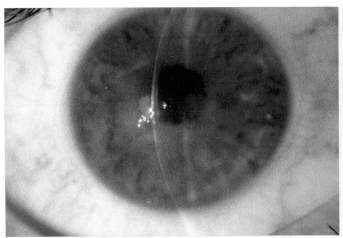

Fig. 13.9 Preoperative appearance of an eye with bullous keratopathy.

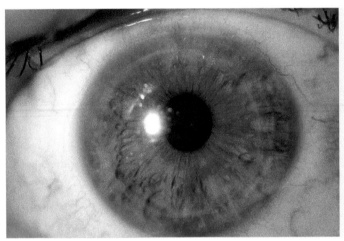

Fig. 13.10 Appearance of the same eye post Descemet's stripping automated endothelial keratoplasty (DSAEK).

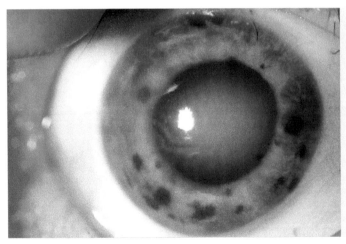

Fig. 13.11 Cataract and corneal decompensation with glaucoma drainage device.

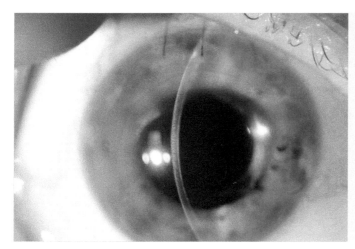

Fig. 13.12 One-week post combined Descemet's stripping automated endothelial keratoplasty (DSAEK) with cataract surgery in the same patient.

DSAEK grafts of a predetermined "UT" thickness and planar profile.[6,39]

The most suitable EK procedure should be considered for each case. Factors determining the best procedure for each eye will include patient factors, surgeon factors, and eye bank factors. Patient factors will include demographics, coexisting ocular pathology, and visual potential. A patient who lives far away or who might struggle to attend follow-up might be better suited to a low-risk procedure such as DSAEK or UT-DSAEK, rather than a procedure with a higher level of complication such as DMEK. Likewise, DSAEK or UT-DSAEK may be better suited to the complex cases such as those requiring concurrent IOL exchange, with glaucoma tubes or shunts, or in aphakic eyes. DMEK might be more appropriate for eyes with excellent visual potential, or those with increased risk of rejection. Surgeon factors are important, especially given the significant learning curve associated with DMEK.[36] Eye bank factors such as availability of precut or prestripped tissue will also be important.

Visual outcomes of EK are in general excellent, with a high proportion of those with visual potential of 20/20 achieving that level within 6 months of surgery, particularly with UT-DSAEK and DMEK.[6,40,41] Patients with bullous keratopathy following cataract surgery can therefore be reassured that EK is an excellent option and that visual recovery is likely.

13.8 Key Pearls

- Bullous keratopathy is a possible cause of suboptimal visual outcome post cataract surgery.

- Preoperative workup includes history, examination, and ancillary tests such as specular microscopy.
- Surgery may be adapted to minimize the endothelial cell loss during cataract surgery in eyes that are at increased risk for development of bullous keratopathy.
- Initial treatment is most often conservative.
- If surgical treatment is required, EK can offer excellent visual outcomes for patients with bullous keratopathy.

References

[1] Eye Bank Association of America. 2015 Eye Banking Statistical Report 2015. Washington, DC: Eye Bank Association of America. Available at: www.restoresight.org. Accessed August 2017
[2] Weiss JS, Møller HU, Lisch W, et al. The IC3D classification of the corneal dystrophies. Cornea. 2008; 27 suppl 2:S1–S83
[3] Wirbelauer C, Anders N, Pham DT, Wollensak J. Corneal endothelial cell changes in pseudoexfoliation syndrome after cataract surgery. Arch Ophthalmol. 1998; 116(2):145–149
[4] Neuhann IM, Neuhann TF, Rohrbach JM. Intraocular lens calcification after keratoplasty. Cornea. 2013; 32(4):e6–e10
[5] Scorcia V, Matteoni S, Scorcia GB, Scorcia G, Busin M. Pentacam assessment of posterior lamellar grafts to explain hyperopization after Descemet's stripping automated endothelial keratoplasty. Ophthalmology. 2009; 116(9):1651–1655
[6] Busin M, Madi S, Santorum P, Scorcia V, Beltz J. Ultrathin descemet's stripping automated endothelial keratoplasty with the microkeratome double-pass technique: two-year outcomes. Ophthalmology. 2013; 120(6):1186–1194
[7] Price MO, Giebel AW, Fairchild KM, Price FW, Jr. Descemet's membrane endothelial keratoplasty: prospective multicenter study of visual and refractive outcomes and endothelial survival. Ophthalmology. 2009; 116(12):2361–2368
[8] Arshinoff SA. Dispersive-cohesive viscoelastic soft shell technique. J Cataract Refract Surg. 1999; 25(2):167–173

[9] Miyata K, Nagamoto T, Maruoka S, Tanabe T, Nakahara M, Amano S. Efficacy and safety of the soft-shell technique in cases with a hard lens nucleus. J Cataract Refract Surg. 2002; 28(9):1546–1550

[10] Kim D-H, Wee W-R, Lee J-H, Kim M-K. The comparison between torsional and conventional mode phacoemulsification in moderate and hard cataracts. Korean J Ophthalmol. 2010; 24(6):336–340

[11] Leon P, Umari I, Mangogna A, Zanei A, Tognetto D. An evaluation of intraoperative and postoperative outcomes of torsional mode versus longitudinal ultrasound mode phacoemulsification: a meta-analysis. Int J Ophthalmol. 2016; 9(6): 890–897

[12] Park J, Yum HR, Kim MS, Harrison AR, Kim EC. Comparison of phaco-chop, divide-and-conquer, and stop-and-chop phaco techniques in microincision coaxial cataract surgery. J Cataract Refract Surg. 2013; 39(10):1463–1469

[13] Khokhar S, Aron N, Sen S, Pillay G, Agarwal E. Effect of balanced phacoemulsification tip on the outcomes of torsional phacoemulsification using an active-fluidics system. J Cataract Refract Surg. 2017; 43(1):22–28

[14] Gogate P, Ambardekar P, Kulkarni S, Deshpande R, Joshi S, Deshpande M. Comparison of endothelial cell loss after cataract surgery: phacoemulsification versus manual small-incision cataract surgery: six-week results of a randomized control trial. J Cataract Refract Surg. 2010; 36 (2):247–253

[15] Bhargava R, Sharma SK, Chandra M, Kumar P, Arora Y. Comparison of endothelial cell loss and complications between phacoemulsification and manual small incision cataract surgery (SICS) in uveitic cataract. Nepal J Ophthalmol. 2015; 7(14):124–134

[16] Zhang JY, Feng YF, Cai JQ. Phacoemulsification versus manual small-incision cataract surgery for age-related cataract: meta-analysis of randomized controlled trials. Clin Experiment Ophthalmol. 2013; 41(4):379–386

[17] Nayak BK, Shukla RO. Effect on corneal endothelial cell loss during phacoemulsification: fortified balanced salt solution versus Ringer lactate. J Cataract Refract Surg. 2012; 38(9): 1552–1558

[18] Lucena DR, Ribeiro MS, Messias A, Bicas HE, Scott IU, Jorge R. Comparison of corneal changes after phacoemulsification using BSS Plus versus Lactated Ringer's irrigating solution: a prospective randomised trial. Br J Ophthalmol. 2011; 95(4): 485–489

[19] Eggeling P, Pleyer U, Hartmann C, Rieck PW. Corneal endothelial toxicity of different lidocaine concentrations. J Cataract Refract Surg. 2000; 26(9):1403–1408

[20] Abell RG, Kerr NM, Vote BJ. Toward zero effective phacoemulsification time using femtosecond laser pretreatment. Ophthalmology. 2013; 120(5):942–948

[21] Conrad-Hengerer I, Al Juburi M, Schultz T, Hengerer FH, Dick HB. Corneal endothelial cell loss and corneal thickness in conventional compared with femtosecond laser-assisted cataract surgery: three-month follow-up. J Cataract Refract Surg. 2013; 39(9):1307–1313

[22] Krarup T, Holm LM, la Cour M, Kjaerbo H. Endothelial cell loss and refractive predictability in femtosecond laser-assisted cataract surgery compared with conventional cataract surgery. Acta Ophthalmol. 2014; 92(7):617–622

[23] Abell RG, Kerr NM, Howie AR, Mustaffa Kamal MA, Allen PL, Vote BJ. Effect of femtosecond laser-assisted cataract surgery on the corneal endothelium. J Cataract Refract Surg. 2014; 40 (11):1777–1783

[24] Chen X, Chen K, He J, Yao K. Comparing the curative effects between femtosecond laser-assisted cataract surgery and conventional phacoemulsification surgery: a meta-analysis. PLoS One. 2016; 11(3):e0152088

[25] Canner JK, Javitt JC, McBean AM. National outcomes of cataract extraction. III. Corneal edema and transplant following inpatient surgery. Arch Ophthalmol. 1992; 110(8): 1137–1142

[26] Bohigian GM, Wexler SA. Complications of retained nuclear fragments in the anterior chamber after phacoemulsification with posterior chamber lens implant. Am J Ophthalmol. 1997; 123(4):546–547

[27] Chan TC, Lam JK, Jhanji V, Li EY. Comparison of outcomes of primary anterior chamber versus secondary scleral-fixated intraocular lens implantation in complicated cataract surgeries. Am J Ophthalmol. 2015; 159(2):221–6.e2

[28] Wirtitsch MG, Findl O, Heinzl H, Drexler W. Effect of dorzolamide hydrochloride on central corneal thickness in humans with cornea guttata. Arch Ophthalmol. 2007; 125 (10):1345–1350

[29] Lee WB, Jacobs DS, Musch DC, Kaufman SC, Reinhart WJ, Shtein RM. Descemet's stripping endothelial keratoplasty: safety and outcomes: a report by the American Academy of Ophthalmology. Ophthalmology. 2009; 116(9):1818–1830

[30] Melles GR, Ong TS, Ververs B, van der Wees J. Descemet membrane endothelial keratoplasty (DMEK). Cornea. 2006; 25(8):987–990

[31] Guerra FP, Anshu A, Price MO, Price FW. Endothelial keratoplasty: fellow eyes comparison of Descemet stripping automated endothelial keratoplasty and Descemet membrane endothelial keratoplasty. Cornea. 2011; 30(12):1382–1386

[32] Tourtas T, Laaser K, Bachmann BO, Cursiefen C, Kruse FE. Descemet membrane endothelial keratoplasty versus descemet stripping automated endothelial keratoplasty. Am J Ophthalmol. 2012; 153(6):1082–90.e2

[33] Guerra FP, Anshu A, Price MO, Giebel AW, Price FW. Descemet's membrane endothelial keratoplasty: prospective study of 1-year visual outcomes, graft survival, and endothelial cell loss. Ophthalmology. 2011; 118(12):2368–2373

[34] Anshu A, Price MO, Price FW, Jr. Risk of corneal transplant rejection significantly reduced with Descemet's membrane endothelial keratoplasty. Ophthalmology. 2012; 119(3): 536–540

[35] Dapena I, Ham L, Netuková M, van der Wees J, Melles GR. Incidence of early allograft rejection after Descemet membrane endothelial keratoplasty. Cornea. 2011; 30(12):1341–1345

[36] Terry MA. Endothelial keratoplasty: why aren't we all doing Descemet membrane endothelial keratoplasty? Cornea. 2012; 31(5):469–471

[37] Neff KD, Biber JM, Holland EJ. Comparison of central corneal graft thickness to visual acuity outcomes in endothelial keratoplasty. Cornea. 2011; 30(4):388–391

[38] Rudolph M, Laaser K, Bachmann BO, Cursiefen C, Epstein D, Kruse FE. Corneal higher-order aberrations after Descemet's membrane endothelial keratoplasty. Ophthalmology. 2012; 119(3):528–535

[39] Villarrubia A, Cano-Ortiz A. Development of a nomogram to achieve ultrathin donor corneal disks for Descemet-stripping automated endothelial keratoplasty. J Cataract Refract Surg. 2015; 41(1):146–151

[40] Dapena I, Ham L, Droutsas K, van Dijk K, Moutsouris K, Melles GR. Learning curve in Descemet's membrane endothelial keratoplasty: first series of 135 consecutive cases. Ophthalmology. 2011; 118(11):2147–2154

[41] Rodríguez-Calvo-de-Mora M, Quilendrino R, Ham L, et al. Clinical outcome of 500 consecutive cases undergoing Descemet's membrane endothelial keratoplasty. Ophthalmology. 2015; 122(3):464–470

14 Malpositioned Intraocular Lens and Capsular Bag: Intraocular Lens Complex Issues

Amar Agarwal

Abstract

Malpositioned intraocular lens (IOL) with capsular bag–IOL complex requires an immediate attention with necessary surgical intervention that may range from an IOL explantation to repositioning or to a secondary IOL fixation. This chapter highlights the issue of IOL tilt, decentration, and malposition that can lead to suboptimal outcomes. The capsular bag–IOL complex issues will also be covered along with the techniques to realign the IOL and manage the case as per surgical scenario.

Keywords: malpositioned IOL, decentration, glued IOL, IOL scaffold, IOL exchange, Subluxation, Repositioning, capsular bag–IOL complex, IOL explant

14.1 Malpositioned Intraocular Lens

14.1.1 Introduction

Malpositioning of an intraocular lens (IOL) may range from mild decentration to complete luxation in the posterior segment. Although the frequency of IOL dislocation ranges from 0.2 to 3%,[1,2,3,4,5,6,7,8,9] clinically insignificant and significant decentrations are seen in 25% and 3% of the cases, respectively.[10,11] Malpositioned IOLs often present with extreme decentration to the extent that the IOL optic covers only a small portion of the pupillary space (▶ Fig. 14.1). Depending on the amount of IOL dislocation, the patient may present with symptoms of decreased vision and associated complications such as cystoid macular edema (CME), vitritis, corneal decompensation, secondary glaucoma, and retinal involvement. IOL malposition or dislocation can occur either in the initial postoperative period or during any phase of the entire postoperative period depending on the causal factor and associated etiology and predisposing factor.

14.1.2 Management

The management of a malpositioned IOL depends on various factors that may range from the timing of onset of dislocation to the etiology and to the extent of dislocation along with the type of the IOL that is malpositioned in the eye. The surgeon needs to make a decision between the surgical repositioning and refixating the same IOL and performing an IOL exchange. In such a situation, the presence of a three-piece IOL in the eye has a distinct advantage as it can be repositioned and placed in the sulcus with or without an optic capture or the haptics of the same IOL can be externalized and tucked into the intrascleral pockets as in a glued intrascleral haptic (glued IOL) fixation[12,13,14,15] in cases with inadequate sulcus support (▶ Fig. 14.2, ▶ Fig. 14.3, ▶ Fig. 14.4).

14.1.3 Repositioning the Intraocular Lens

Repositioning, if possible, has a distinct advantage of closed chamber approach with the appropriate surgical alignment of the IOL. The amount of maneuver needed to reposition the IOL depends on the type of the IOL and the associated condition in the eye. In cases with inappropriately dialed IOL where one haptic lies in the capsular bag and the other haptic is outside the capsular bag, a simple intervention of inflating the capsular bag and the anterior chamber (AC) with an ophthalmic viscosurgical device (OVD) followed by dialing an IOL completely into the capsular bag suffices the need for any further intervention.

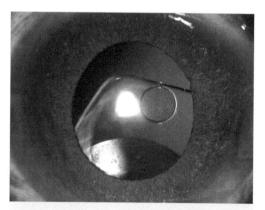

Fig. 14.1 Significantly decentered plate haptic intraocular lens (IOL) with the optic not visualized in the pupillary zone.

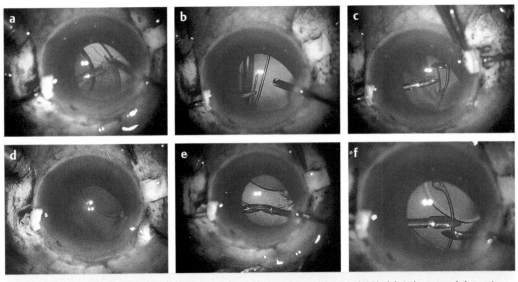

Fig. 14.2 Decentered three-piece intraocular lens (IOL) with capsular tension ring (CTR). (a) A decentered three-piece IOL with a CTR and the entire bag is seen. (b) Two partial-thickness scleral flaps are made 180 degrees opposite along with sclerotomy as in a glued IOL procedure. One IOL haptic is grasped and vitrectomy is performed to cut down all vitreous adhesions and capsular fibrosis. (c) Total cortical and capsular cleanup is achieved. Handshake technique is performed wherein the haptic is transferred from one hand to another for easy haptic externalization and the tip of the haptic is grasped. (d) The tip of the haptic is externalized from the respective sclerotomy site. (e) The CTR is grasped and the handshake technique is performed to reach the tip of the CTR. (f) The handshake technique being performed for CTR.

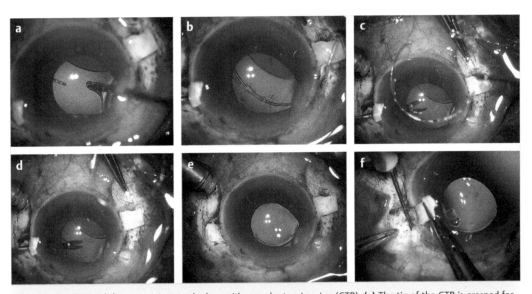

Fig. 14.3 Decentered three-piece intraocular lens with capsular tension ring (CTR). (a) The tip of the CTR is grasped for externalization. (b) The CTR is pulled from the corneal incision. (c) The CTR is removed. (d) The externalized haptic is grasped with an end-opening forceps. (e) Both the haptics are externalized. (f) Scleral pockets are created with a 26-gauge needle.

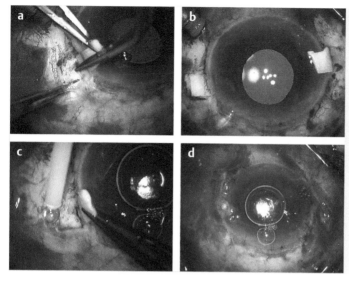

Fig. 14.4 Decentered three-piece intraocular lens with capsular tension ring (CTR). **(a)** Haptic tucked into the scleral pockets. **(b)** Both haptics are tucked into the scleral pockets. **(c)** Fibrin glue is applied beneath the flaps. **(d)** The scleral flaps and the conjunctival incisions are sealed with fibrin glue. The corneal tunnel incision is closed with a 10–0 suture and air bubble is put into the anterior chamber.

Decentration may be associated with a posterior capsule rupture (PCR) and in these cases the type of IOL present in the eye plays the key decision maker along with the surgical technique that the surgeon is most comfortable employing in such a demanding condition.

Presence of One-Piece Intraocular Lens

In cases with intraoperative PCR, often after vitrectomy in a localized small posterior capsule (PC) tear, surgeons place a one-piece foldable IOL in the capsular bag. Although this suffices the need at that hour, in late postoperative follow-up period decentrations have been reported to occur. An initial attempt at vitrectomy from the pars plana route allows cutting all the vitreous behind the IOL and the capsular bag. Decompressing the posterior chamber helps obviate the push from behind the IOL and helps stabilize the capsular bag. After adequate vitrectomy, the IOL can be dialed again in its position and if possible optic capture can be attempted although it is a bit difficult to capture a one-piece IOL. In cases with massive PCR with decentration of one-piece IOL, the surgeon is left with the only option of IOL explantation.

Presence of a Three-Piece Intraocular Lens

Ideally in cases of PCR, a three-piece IOL should always be placed either in the bag or in the sulcus.

Doing so has an added advantage that in cases of decentrations, the IOL can be easily and safely repositioned either in the sulcus or in the bag, thereby minimizing the chances of an IOL exchange (▶ Fig. 14.2, ▶ Fig. 14.3, ▶ Fig. 14.4).

14.1.4 Intraocular Lens Exchange/Explant

Decentrations and malpositioned IOLs call for surgical intervention when repositioning does not suffice the need. The type of IOL to be reimplanted in the eye depends on the etiology of the decentration.

In cases with either damage to the IOL at the optic haptic junction or with cut haptics, the IOL needs to be explanted and exchanged. An IOL of the same type can be placed in the bag, as the cause of decentration was IOL damage. However, in cases with multifocal IOL intolerance, the multifocal IOL needs to be exchanged for a monofocal IOL.

In cases of decentration with associated PCR, the one-piece IOL if present is explanted, followed by placement of a three-piece IOL in the sulcus with/without an optic capture.

Intraocular Lens Scaffold for Intraocular Lens Exchange

In this technique,[16] the offending IOL is manipulated out of the capsular bag into the AC, and the corrective IOL is inserted into the bag.

With Intact Posterior Capsule

The offending IOL is levitated from the bag and is brought into the AC. A new corrective IOL is then injected into the AC beneath the offending IOL. The corrective IOL is then dialed into the capsular bag and is placed in position. The anteriorly elevated IOL is transected with the IOL cutting scissors, while the corrective IOL acts as a scaffold for the PC. The offending IOL is cut with IOL cutting scissors and is then explanted out of the AC. The continuous distension of the bag with the presence of the IOL prevents damage to the PC while the IOL is being cut.

With Broken Posterior Capsule

Through pars plana approach, a limited vitrectomy is performed beneath the capsular opening and the IOL is then levitated into the AC from the limbal approach. A corrective IOL is then dialed into the capsular bag in a way that it plugs the posterior capsular opening altogether and also acts as a barrier to vitreous prolapse in cases of an open PC. This method works effectively in cases with small PC openings only as in cases where a previous yttrium aluminum garnet (Yag) capsulotomy has been performed. The offending IOL is then cut and explanted. The corrective IOL is always a three-piece IOL so that in cases with further issues with decentration, the IOL can be refixated with the glued technique[12,13,14,15] or it can be placed in the sulcus if feasible.

In cases involving IOL exchange from a capsule fixated IOL many months or years postoperatively, the surgeon should carefully open the capsular bag and successfully use the scaffold technique to protect the PC or avoid vitreous prolapse if the PC is open. Adequate caution should be exercised while dialing the IOL haptic out of the capsular bag to avoid undue stress on the capsule.

In cases of complete loss of capsular support along with IOL decentration, the IOL needs to be explanted altogether and secondary IOL implantation is the only choice that the surgeon is left with. A scleral tunnel incision is framed and often the author prefers to adopt the "**L**"-shaped incision instead of a linear scleral incision as these "**L**"-shaped incisions are considered to be astigmatically neutral. For creating an "**L**" tunnel, a 3-mm mark is set on the vernier caliper and the "**L**"-shaped scleral incision is marked (▶ Fig. 14.5a). The crescent blade is used to make the tunnel along the **L**-shaped mark and the tunnel is widened anteriorly and to the sides (intrascleral aspect) creating a nearly 6-mm-wide tunnel (▶ Fig. 14.5b,c,d). An L-shaped incision provides good chamber stability and an equal ease of IOL explantation and insertion from the "**L**" design incision with the added advantage of a good intrascleral extension of the **L**-shaped tunnel incision that facilitates the IOL manipulation. A square incision wherein the length and the width of the incision are equal is the most astigmatically stable wound. **L**-shaped incision has been considered to be superior to the conventional linear incision due to its astigmatic neutral wound architecture. The scar tissue according to Drew's theory tends to contract along its horizontal axis as much as to its perpendicular axis.

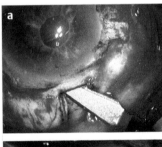
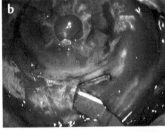
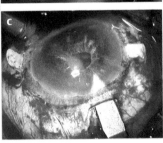
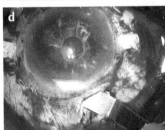

Fig. 14.5 "L"-shaped incision for decentered intraocular lens (IOL) explantation. (a) A 3 × 3 mm mark is made with a vernier caliper in the shape of an "L." Two partial-thickness scleral flaps made for glued IOL procedure. (b) Crescent blade is used to dissect the tunnel in an "L"-shaped manner. The intrascleral pocket of 3 mm allows the IOL to be explanted as its 6 mm in horizontal dimension. (c) A keratome opens the incision. (d) The keratome extends the intrascleral portion of the "L"-shaped incision that provides a valvular effect.

Once the IOL is explanted, a three-piece IOL is introduced into the eye (▶ Fig. 14.6) and the leading haptic is grasped with a glued IOL forceps and the haptic is externalized. The trailing haptic is then introduced inside the eye and the handshake technique is performed, followed by externalization of the haptic from the other sclerotomy site. The haptics are then tucked into the intrascleral pockets created with a 26-gauge needle, followed by vitrectomy at the sclerotomy sites. Fibrin glue is applied and the flaps are sealed along with all the conjunctival wounds.

14.1.5 Sleeveless Extrusion Cannula-Assisted Levitation for Dropped IOL

Dr. Ashvin Agarwal started this technique in which the sleeve of the extrusion cannula is removed before managing the dropped IOL (▶ Fig. 14.7). Removal of the silicon sleeve exposes wider access of the bore of the cannula, which helps create an effective suction around the IOL.[17]

In this technique, after adequate vitrectomy the sleeveless-extrusion cannula is connected to the

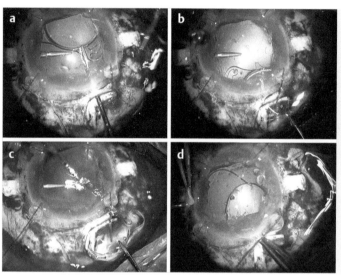

Fig. 14.6 "L"-shaped incision for decentered intraocular lens (IOL) explantation. **(a)** The one-piece IOL is grasped with an end-opening forceps introduced from the incision. Iris hooks are placed in position to widen the pupillary aperture and enhance the visualization. **(b)** The IOL being explanted. **(c)** The IOL is explanted totally. **(d)** A three-piece IOL being introduced in to the eye for glued IOL fixation.

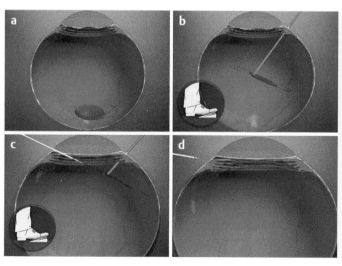

Fig. 14.7 Extrusion cannula assisted levitation of dropped intraocular lens (IOL). **(a)** The dropped IOL lying on the retina. **(b)** Sleeveless extrusion cannula creates suction on the optic of the IOL. **(c)** The dropped IOL is lifted and brought into the pupillary plane and is grasped with an end-opening forceps. **(d)** The IOL is placed on to the sulcus support if present or is explanted as per the surgical scenario.

vitreotome and the vacuum is set to 300 mm Hg with the cutting function turned off. As the IOL rests flat on the retina, the sleeveless extrusion cannula is made to face the center of the optic and suction is initiated, which can be dynamically controlled with the foot pedal. The linear control of the foot pedal helps increase the vacuum as and when needed during the levitation of IOL. Ineffective apposition of the lumen of the cannula to the surface of the IOL optic can lead to loss of vacuum. The IOL is lifted from the surface of the retina and is brought into the anterior vitreous in the midpupillary area. The end-opening forceps introduced from the corneal incision under direct visualization through the microscope grasp the IOL; the extrusion cannula is then removed as the forceps grasp the IOL. The IOL can then be subsequently managed depending on the surgical scenario. It can be either replaced or repositioned in the sulcus or explanted.

The advantage with this technique is that it is safe, reliable, and reproducible. Moreover, it is effective for dislocation of any type of IOL including the plate haptic IOLs, which are often difficult to grasp with a retinal forceps.

14.2 Capsular Bag–IOL Complex Issues

Secured in the capsular bag–IOL placement is the most desirable outcome of postcataract surgery although decentrations of the capsular bag due to either zonular compromise or shrinkage of the capsular bag are a known entity. The IOL may be securely placed in the capsular bag, but the bag itself may decenter leading to IOL decentration and in extreme cases luxation where the entire bag–IOL complex may be lying in the vitreous cavity. Often due to shrinkage of capsular bag, the IOL folds upon itself, leading to further shrinkage and contraction of the capsular bag. Capsular tension rings (CTRs) are implanted into the capsular bag with the intention of distending the bag and preventing the shrinkage in predisposed cases with pseudoexfoliation, uveitis, myopia, and other connective tissue disorders that affect the zonular stability. Despite this, the capsular bag dislocations are encountered and need to be managed effectively.[18,19]

14.2.1 Management of Subluxated/Dislocated Bag–IOL Complex

The presence of a partially subluxated bag–IOL complex can be handled through an anterior segment approach if the bag–IOL complex is in the pupillary zone. A scleral tunnel or a limbal approach can be adopted and the bag–IOL complex can be levitated into the AC followed by its explantation. After performing thorough vitrectomy, secondary IOL fixation should be considered in these cases. A total dislocation of the capsular bag–IOL complex into the vitreous cavity calls for a posterior segment approach by a vitreoretinal surgeon (▶ Fig. 14.8). After performing vitrectomy and removal of all adhesions around the bag–IOL complex, it can be levitated in to the AC and managed subsequently. Glued IOL fixation can be done in these cases with a three-piece foldable IOL being trans-sclerally fixed and placed in position.

In cases with a three-piece IOL being present in the dislocated bag–IOL complex (▶ Fig. 14.9a, b), the complex can be held with an end-opening forceps and all the adhesions around the IOL can be cut with the vitrectomy probe. Once the IOL is freed from all the adhesions, the haptics can be externalized from the sclerotomy openings as in a glued IOL surgery (▶ Fig. 14.9c–e). The haptics are then tucked into the scleral pockets created with a 26-gauge needle (▶ Fig. 14.9f) followed by sealing

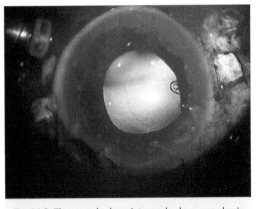

Fig. 14.8 The capsular bag–intraocular lens complex is completely luxated in to the vitreous cavity.

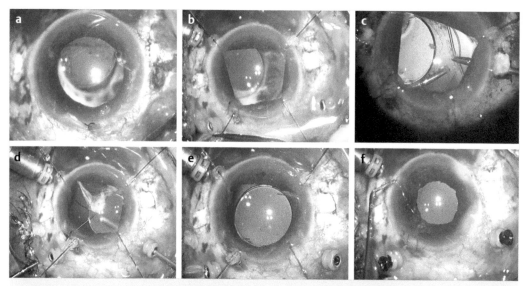

Fig. 14.9 Subluxated capsular bag–intraocular lens (IOL) complex in a case of pseudoexfoliation. **(a)** The endocapsular segment is seen dislodged into the anterior chamber in a case of subluxated capsular bag–IOL complex. **(b)** The endocapsular segment is explanted through the corneal incision and the wound is secured with 10–0 suture. Iris hooks are employed for adequate visualization and standard three-port pars plana trocars are placed in position. **(c)** The capsular bag–IOL complex is held with an end-opening forceps and thorough vitrectomy is performed to clean up all the adhesions around the IOL. A capsular tension ring (CTR) is also seen to be placed in the bag. **(d)** The haptics are externalized and the CTR is held and all adhesions around it are cut followed by its explantation. **(e)** Both haptics externalized from the sclerotomy sites beneath the scleral flaps. **(f)** The haptics are tucked into the scleral pockets and all incisions are sealed. A well-centered IOL is seen.

of the flaps and the conjunctival wounds with the fibrin glue application.

Various techniques have been described for refixating the bag–IOL complex to the scleral wall and to the iris tissue with sutures.[20,21,22,23] This method has an added advantage of having a closed chamber approach without the need for enlarging an incision, thereby minimizing the surgically induced astigmatism and the vitreous prolapse. Surgeons usually choose a 9–0 Prolene over the 10–0 Prolene suture although degradation of suture has been reported with both 9–0 and 10–0 sutures. Suture degradation can lead to decentrations again (▶ Fig. 14.10) and the IOL may have to be explanted again (▶ Fig. 14.10, ▶ Fig. 14.11, ▶ Fig. 14.12) depending on the severity of the condition. GORE-TEX suture is currently the preferred choice of surgeons, as it is believed to be nondegradable and thus can last longer.

14.3 Discussion

In the management of dislocated or malpositioned IOLs, a decision needs to be made with regard to whether an IOL exchange or IOL repositioning

should be performed along with the route of approach. With the various permutations and combinations that the clinical scenario may offer, the surgeon choses the method of approach and surgical tackling of the case. The type of IOL present in the eye also plays a key role in deciding the approach that can be adopted in handling the case effectively. The optic diameter, the IOL configuration, type of haptics, and the IOL material present help define the further status. Regardless of all the factors, the most essential consideration in these cases is handling the vitreous and minimizing its disturbance to avoid subsequent inflammatory and tractional complications.

Surgical repair should be considered in cases with substantial loss of vision following a dislocated or a malpositioned IOL. Although the frequency of clinically significant IOL dislocation is low, a carefully guided approach may help optimize the outcomes of this complication.

14.4 Key Pearls

- Mild decentrations of the IOL that do not cause any visual symptom can be followed up without

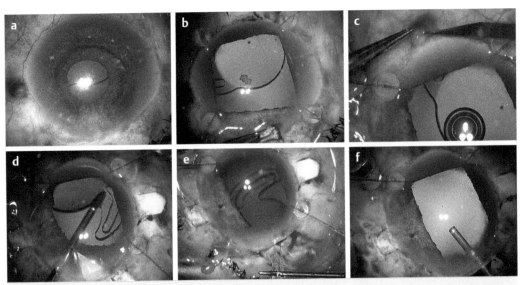

Fig. 14.10 Decentered sutured intraocular lens (IOL). **(a)** A decentered IOL with the optic covering the midpupillary area is seen. **(b)** Two scleral flaps for glued IOL are made and iris hooks are employed. **(c)** The suture at one end of the haptic is held and is cut to free the IOL as the other end of suture had already degraded. **(d)** A scleral tunnel incision is made and the IOL is held with an end-opening forceps. **(e)** The IOL is explanted. **(f)** Adequate thorough vitrectomy is performed.

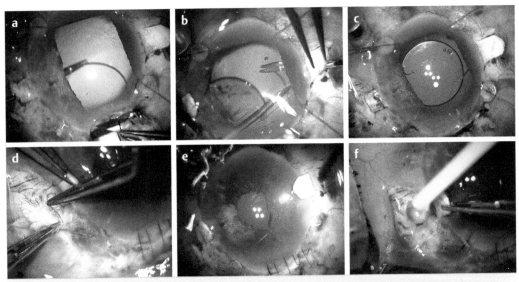

Fig. 14.11 Glued intraocular lens (IOL) fixation following IOL explantation. **(a)** A three-piece IOL introduced in the eye is held with an end-opening glued IOL forceps introduced from the sclerotomy site. **(b)** The leading haptic is externalized and the trailing haptic is introduced inside the eye. The tip of the trailing haptic is held with glued IOL forceps introduced from the right sclerotomy site. **(c)** Both the haptics are externalized. **(d)** Haptic being tucked into the scleral pocket. **(e)** Both haptics tucked into the scleral pockets. **(f)** Scleral flaps being sealed with fibrin glue.

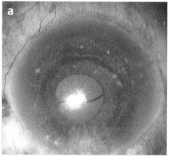 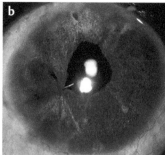

Fig. 14.12 Pre- and postoperative images. **(a)** Preoperative image of a case with decentered intraocular lens (IOL). **(b)** Postoperative image at 2 months. IOL explantation was done and secondary IOL implantation with glued IOL fixation technique was performed. A well-centered IOL is seen covering the entire pupil.

any active surgical intervention, whereas symptomatic decentrations need a surgical correction.

- Repositioning of an IOL should be considered if stable fixation can be achieved or else an IOL exchange should be performed.
- A vitreoretinal associate should handle the dislocation of IOL or the bag–IOL complex in to the midvitreous cavity and beyond, and fishing movement into the vitreous cavity should be avoided.
- A three-piece subluxated IOL can be refixated with a closed chamber technique with glued intrascleral haptic fixation of an IOL.
- A one-piece IOL should never be repositioned or placed into the sulcus. A three-piece IOL suffices the need of safe sulcus placement of an IOL.

Videos

Video 14.1 L-shaped pocket incision and subluxated one-piece intraocular lens (IOL). The subluxated one-piece IOL is explanted through an L-shaped scleral incision that is considered astigmatically neutral. A three-piece IOL is fixed with the glued intrascleral fixation technique.

Video 14.2 Subluxated one-piece foldable intraocular lens (IOL) with single-pass four-throw (SFT) pupilloplasty. With fluid infusion inside the eye, a scleral tunnel is made. The tunnel is enlarged and the single-piece foldable IOL is explanted. A new three-piece foldable IOL is then fixated inside the eye. Pupilloplasty is performed with the SFT technique to prevent optic capture in the postoperative period.

Video 14.3 Subluxated intraocular lens (IOL) with broken haptics. Vertical flaps are made at the 12 and 6 o'clock positions. The subluxated IOL is found to be sutured with the scleral wall and the iris. The adhesions are cut and the IOL is

released. The broken haptic and the IOL are explanted from the scleral tunnel incision. Glued IOL fixation is then performed with a three-piece IOL followed by SFT pupilloplasty.

Video 14.4 Subluxated anterior chamber intraocular lens (ACIOL) with haptic protrusion in the sclera. The ACIOL is explanted and all the adhesions are cut in the AC, followed by glued IOL fixation. Pupil repair is done by the single-pass four-throw (SFT) pupilloplasty procedure.

Video 14.5 Malpositioned three-piece intraocular lens (IOL) in sulcus. After thorough vitrectomy, refixation of the same subluxated IOL is done with glued IOL technique. (This video is provided courtesy of Priya Narang.)

Video 14.6 Dropped intraocular lens (IOL). The various aspects of handling a dropped IOL along with vitrectomy and secondary IOL implantation are described in detail.

References

[1] Taylor DM, Dalburg LA, Consentino RT, Khaliq A. Intraocular lenses: 500 consecutive intracapsular cataract extractions with lens implantation compared with 500 intracapsular extractions—observations and comments. Ophthalmic Surg. 1978; 9(1):29–55

[2] Kratz RP. Complications associated with posterior chamber lenses. Ophthalmology. 1979; 86(4):659–661

[3] Worthen DM, Boucher JA, Buxton JN, et al. Interim FDA report on intraocular lenses. Ophthalmology. 1980; 87(4): 267–271

[4] Kratz RP, Mazzocco TR, Davidson B, Colvard DM. The Shearing intraocular lens: a report of 1,000 cases. J Am Intraocul Implant Soc. 1981; 7(1):55–57

[5] Jaffe NS, Clayman HM, Jaffe MS, Light DS. The results of extracapsular cataract extraction with a shearing posterior chamber lens implant 34 to 40 months after surgery. Ophthalmic Surg. 1982; 13(1):47–49

[6] Stark WJ, Worthen DM, Holladay JT, et al. The FDA report on intraocular lenses. Ophthalmology. 1983; 90(4):311–317

[7] Kraff MC, Sanders DR, Lieberman HL. The results of posterior chamber lens implantation. J Am Intraocul Implant Soc. 1983; 9(2):148–150

[8] Southwick PC, Olson RJ. Shearing posterior chamber intraocular lenses: five-year postoperative results. J Am Intraocul Implant Soc. 1984; 10(3):318–323

[9] Smith SG, Lindstrom RL. Malpositioned posterior chamber lenses: etiology, prevention, and management. J Am Intraocul Implant Soc. 1985; 11(6):584–591

[10] Pallin SL, Walman GB. Posterior chamber intraocular lens implant centration: in or out of "the bag". Am Intra-Ocular Implant Soc J.. 1982; 8:254–257

[11] Böke WR, Krüger HCA. Causes and management of posterior chamber lens displacement. J Am Intraocul Implant Soc. 1985; 11(2):179–184

[12] Agarwal A, Kumar DA, Jacob S, Baid C, Agarwal A, Srinivasan S. Fibrin glue-assisted sutureless posterior chamber intraocular lens implantation in eyes with deficient posterior capsules. J Cataract Refract Surg. 2008; 34(9):1433–1438

[13] Narang P, Narang S. Glue-assisted intrascleral fixation of posterior chamber intraocular lens. Indian J Ophthalmol. 2013; 61(4):163–167

[14] Narang P. Modified method of haptic externalization of posterior chamber intraocular lens in fibrin glue-assisted intrascleral fixation: no-assistant technique. J Cataract Refract Surg. 2013; 39(1):4–7

[15] Narang P, Agarwal A. Peripheral iridectomy for atraumatic haptic externalization in large eyes having anterior sclerotomy for glued intraocular lens. J Cataract Refract Surg. 2016; 42(1):3–6

[16] Narang P, Steinert R, Little B, Agarwal A. Intraocular lens scaffold to facilitate intraocular lens exchange. J Cataract Refract Surg. 2014; 40(9):1403–1407

[17] Agarwal A, Narang P, Agarwal A, Kumar DA. Sleeveless-extrusion cannula for levitation of dislocated intraocular lens. Br J Ophthalmol. 2014; 98(7):910–914

[18] Lim MC, Jap AHE, Wong EYM. Surgical management of late dislocated lens capsular bag with intraocular lens and endocapsular tension ring. J Cataract Refract Surg. 2006; 32(3):533–535

[19] Gimbel HV, Condon GP, Kohnen T, Olson RJ, Halkiadakis I. Late in-the-bag intraocular lens dislocation: incidence, prevention, and management. J Cataract Refract Surg. 2005; 31(11):2193–2204

[20] Nakashizuka H, Shimada H, Iwasaki Y, Matsumoto Y, Sato Y. Pars plana suture fixation for intraocular lenses dislocated into the vitreous cavity using a closed-eye cow-hitch technique. J Cataract Refract Surg. 2004; 30(2):302–306

[21] Kokame GT, Yamamoto I, Mandel H. Scleral fixation of dislocated posterior chamber intraocular lenses: Temporary haptic externalization through a clear corneal incision. J Cataract Refract Surg. 2004; 30(5):1049–1056

[22] Oshika T. Transscleral suture fixation of a subluxated posterior chamber lens within the capsular bag. J Cataract Refract Surg. 1997; 23(9):1421–1424

[23] Chan CK, Agarwal A, Agarwal S, Agarwal A. Management of dislocated intraocular implants. Ophthalmol Clin North Am. 2001; 14(4):681–693

15 Posterior Capsular Rupture and Intraocular Lens Implantation

Priya Narang

Abstract

Posterior capsule rupture (PCR) is a dreaded complication of cataract surgery that is often associated with nonemulsified nuclear fragments and often with sinking nucleus that may advance into a dropped nucleus if not managed properly. The chapter highlights the techniques to restrain the extension of PCR and effective placement of an intraocular lens. Various techniques to levitate the nucleus and emulsify the lenticular fragments are also explained in detail with graphic and pictorial images.

Keywords: posterior capsule rupture, vitrectomy, three-piece IOL, triumvirate technique, glued IOL, glued IOL scaffold, IOL scaffold, posterior assisted levitation, modified PAL, trocar-ACM

15.1 Introduction

Posterior capsule rupture (PCR) is an infrequent but a known complication of cataract surgery and it can also be iatrogenically induced during a vitreoretinal surgery.[1,2,3] PCR can lead to significant ocular morbidity and suboptimal outcomes with permanent vision loss if not handled judiciously. Recognition of an intraoperative PCR in early stages is extremely important to limit the extent of complication and prevent it from being detrimental to a greater extent.

Loss of followability of the nuclear fragments, sudden deepening of the anterior chamber (AC) with pupil dilation, and sudden appearance of red glow are some of the early signs of a PCR. At this stage, the surgeon should lower down the machine parameters and try to assess the clinical scenario. Before the phacoemulsification probe is withdrawn from the eye, ophthalmic viscosurgical device (OVD) is injected into the AC from the side port incision. This helps prevent sudden shallowing of the AC and further extension of the PCR. Subsequent to PCR, the initial objective is the safe and thorough removal of vitreous and lens fragments from the AC, followed by the next prime objective of the stable placement of an intraocular lens (IOL) selected for best refractive outcomes.

Newer techniques available to anterior and posterior segment surgeons in the setting of PCR allow the surgeons to manage the nuclear fragments with the simultaneous placement of an IOL that acts as scaffold and can be used as a pupillary barrier that blocks the subsequent drop of nuclear fragment into the vitreous cavity during its removal through phacoemulsification.

15.2 Management

The management of PCR depends on the stage at which the PCR occurred and also on the extent of posterior capsule opening. PCR in the initial stages of surgery entails the management of entire nucleus/nuclear fragments along with the vitreous and PC opening management, whereas in the later stages it involves the managing the cortical matter and the vitreous prolapse (▶ Fig. 15.1). Often, with big posterior capsule opening, nucleus drop also may occur that involves the management from a vitreoretinal surgeon.

15.3 Vitrectomy and Its Importance

Disruption of the anterior vitreoretinal barrier can enhance the rate of postoperative complications such as endophthalmitis, retinal detachment, and

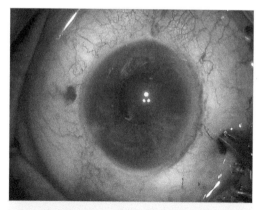

Fig. 15.1 Posterior capsule rupture with residual cortical matter.

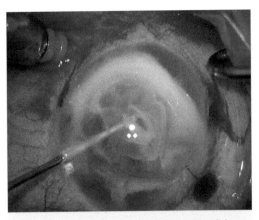

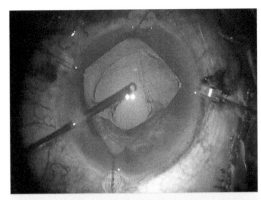

Fig. 15.4 Vitrectomy being performed after pupil dilation with iris hooks.

Fig. 15.2 Triamcinolone staining for detection of the vitreous strands in anterior chamber.

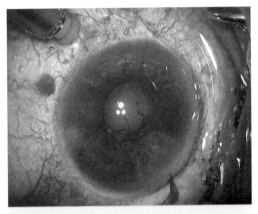

Fig. 15.3 Fluid infusion is introduced into the eye to perform vitrectomy.

cystoid macular edema.[4,5] Along with this, complete removal of the vitreous from the AC is equally essential as it can lead to traction and it can also be detrimental to the corneal endothelium along with the raise of intraocular pressure (IOP). Staining of the transparent vitreous can help a lot in optimizing the visual outcomes as the stained vitreous strands can be easily visualized and managed by the surgeon.[6,7,8]

Triamcinolone staining (▶ Fig. 15.2) is the most common method employed for enhancing the visualization of the prolapsed vitreous.[9,10] Triamcinolone acetonide aids in the visualization of transparent ocular structures by attachment to the collagen matrix of vitreous.[11,12] Before starting anterior vitrectomy, triamcinolone acetonide can be instilled into the AC. This enhances the visibility

of vitreous and ensures adequate vitreous cutting with the vitrector along with appropriate judgment of the endpoint of vitrectomy.

Introduction of infusion into the eye is essential (▶ Fig. 15.3, ▶ Fig. 15.4) before performing vitrectomy. The basic principle of vitreous cutting should be adopted. "Cutting should be more than suction." In other words, the vitrectomy cutter rate should be set higher, whereas the suction should be at moderate levels because if we do not follow this rule and have suction rate more than the cutting rate, then a lot of vitreous gets aspirated even before the vitreous strands have been completely cut. This can lead to vitreous traction and all its sequential complications.

15.4 Posterior Assisted Levitation

Packard and Kinnear described the technique of levitating the sinking nucleus with a spatula[13] that was later named as posterior assisted levitation (PAL) by Kelman.[14,15] Chang and Packard[16] described Viscoat-assisted PAL where through the pars plana site a Viscoat filled cannula is introduced and the Viscoat is injected beneath the nucleus so that it helps cushion the nuclear fragments that are then lifted with the cannula of the Viscoat-filled syringe into the AC.

Following a PCR, the corneal tunnel incision is sutured, as it is essential to secure the wound. The sclerotomy incision for PAL can be made with a micro-vitreoretinal blade or with a trocar at a distance of 3 to 3.5 mm away from the limbus in the

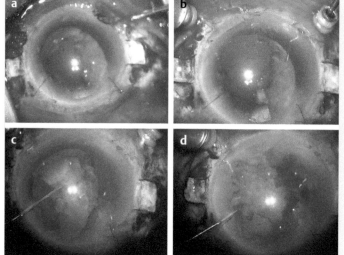

Fig. 15.5 Posterior assisted levitation. (a) Nuclear fragment seen lying in the pupillary zone. (b) Standard pars plana incision made with trocar. A rod is inserted through the trocar to lift the nucleus. (c) The rod is placed beneath the nuclear fragment and the nuclear pieces are pushed forward and placed into the anterior chamber (AC). Another rod inserted from the side port incision can be used to support the nuclear pieces that are being levitated into the AC. (d) All the nuclear pieces are resting into the AC.

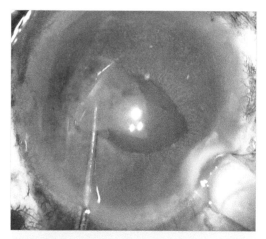

Fig. 15.6 An intraocular lens scaffold procedure where the nucleus is levitated into anterior chamber.

region of pars plana. Trocars have an advantage of creating a self-sealing incision without the need of conjunctival peritomy.

A rod is passed through the trocar and the nuclear fragments are manipulated and lifted with the rod into the AC (▶ Fig. 15.5a, b). While doing PAL, another rod can also be passed from the side port incision so as to support the fragments when they are present in the AC and prevent them from falling back into the vitreous cavity (▶ Fig. 15.5c, d). Once the fragments are in the AC, they are made to rest on the anterior surface of the iris tissue.

15.5 Intraocular Lens Scaffold

The word scaffold is derived from Medieval Latin word "*scaffuldus*" of Old French origin, which means "a temporary platform." As the name suggests, an IOL is used as a scaffold to compartmentalize the eye into anterior and posterior segments with the placement of an IOL that seals the posterior capsular opening.[17,18]

As soon as the PCR is recognized, the surgery is halted and OVD is injected from the side port incision to stabilize the AC. The phaco probe is then withdrawn and all the nuclear fragments are levitated into the AC (▶ Fig. 15.6). A trocar or an AC maintainer (ACM) is introduced into the eye and fluid is switched ON with care being taken that the flow of fluid does not push the nuclear pieces into the vitreous cavity. A limited vitrectomy is done at moderate settings and a three-piece foldable IOL is injected beneath the nuclear fragments. The haptics are made to rest either on the anterior surface of the iris tissue or in the sulcus above the margin of capsulorhexis. Phacoemulsification probe is then introduced and the remaining nuclear fragments are emulsified with phaco machine set at low parameters (▶ Fig. 15.7).

Once the nuclear fragments are emulsified (▶ Fig. 15.8), the IOL is dialed into the sulcus if placed previously on the iris tissue. With the preplacement of an IOL, a barrier is created between the AC and the posterior chamber. The IOL also prevents the nucleus drop and also facilitates emulsification procedure by acting as a scaffold.

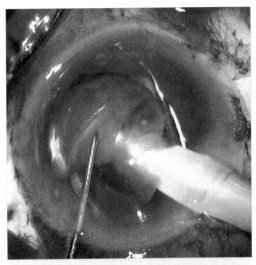

Fig. 15.7 A three-piece foldable intraocular lens is injected beneath the nuclear fragments and is placed above the iris tissue. The nucleus is emulsified with a phaco probe.

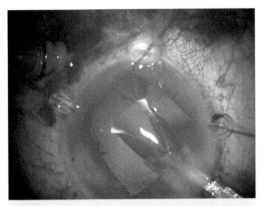

Fig. 15.9 A three-piece foldable intraocular lens is being placed into the sulcus.

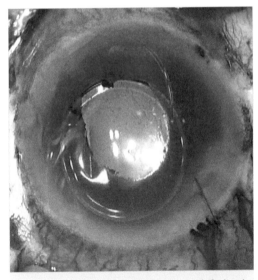

Fig. 15.8 All the nuclear fragments are emulsified and the intraocular lens (IOL) is seen resting on the anterior surface of the iris tissue. This IOL is then dialed into the sulcus.

IOL scaffold allows the management of PCR without enlargement of the corneal incision, thereby passing all the advantages of a closed chamber incision surgery.

The limitation with this technique is that it cannot be adopted for very hard cataract as the nucleus is emulsified in AC close to the corneal endothelium and doing so can lead to damage to the corneal endothelial cell count. Due precaution should be taken while performing IOL scaffold and it is recommended to coat the endothelium with adequate amount of OVD. In cases with dilated pupil, the optic haptic junction can be manipulated with the dialer so as to block the pupillary aperture with the IOL optic during nuclear emulsification in order to prevent any nuclear fragment from slipping into the vitreous cavity.

15.6 Optic Capture

Once the nuclear fragments are emulsified, optic capture as a procedure can be performed to stabilize the IOL placement in cases with adequate sulcus support and good continuous curvilinear capsulorhexis (CCC). The essentials for performing an optic capture are a capsulorhexis that is at least 1 to 2 mm smaller than the diameter of the IOL so that the CCC opening gets plugged by the IOL optic, thereby preventing the vitreous from bulging into the AC. Gimbel and DeBroff[19] have described six different types of optic capture that can be employed by the surgeons for stable IOL placement in cases with PCR. The different variations are as follows:

1. Both haptics in the sulcus and IOL optic capture through anterior CCC (▶ Fig. 15.9, ▶ Fig. 15.10, ▶ Fig. 15.11).
2. Both haptics in the sulcus and IOL optic capture through an anterior capsule opening and a posterior CCC (PCCC).

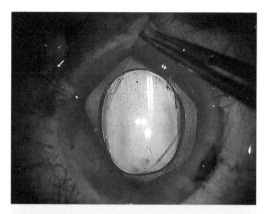

Fig. 15.10 The intraocular lens is dialed into the sulcus with the optic capture into the margins of anterior capsulorhexis.

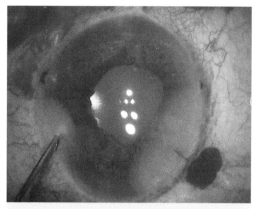

Fig. 15.11 A well-tucked intraocular lens into the sulcus with optic capture. Corneal incisions are sutured with 10–0 nylon.

3. Both haptics in the capsular bag and IOL optic capture through a PCCC.
4. Both haptics in the capsular bag and IOL optic capture through an anterior CCC.
5. Both haptics in the sulcus and IOL capture through a capsular membrane opening.
6. Both haptics posterior to the capsular bag and IOL capture through a capsular membrane opening.

Although all the variations can be applied clinically, out of all the variations described, variations 1, 3, and 4 are the most commonly employed variations. A three-piece foldable IOL is preferable to perform optic capture as compared to one-piece IOL as polypropylene haptics provide better stability and it is easy to capture the optic of a three-piece IOL.

Prolapsing the optic anteriorly brings it closer to the iris and increases the risk for iris chafing and pigment dispersion. If the defect is extremely large or the edges of the posterior capsule defect are not visualized, the posterior chamber IOL haptics should be placed in the ciliary sulcus (with posterior optic capture through an intact anterior capsulorhexis). In cases of posterior capsule tear during or after posterior chamber IOL insertion, leaving the haptics in the capsular bag, rather than trying to dial them out into the sulcus, minimizes vitreous disturbance.

15.7 Glued Intraocular Lens

Glued intrascleral haptic fixation (glued IOL) is an established technique for secondary IOL fixation.[20,21,22,23] Two partial-thickness scleral flaps approximately 2×2 mm are made 180 degrees opposite to each other. Sclerotomy is done with a 22-gauge needle about 1 mm from the limbus beneath the scleral flaps. After the introduction of infusion in the eye, thorough vitrectomy is done to clear the vitreous in the pupillary space and the AC. An ACM or a trocar-ACM[24] can be employed for fluid infusion into the AC or trocar can also be placed at pars plana site depending on the surgeon's preference. A 23-gauge vitrectomy probe is introduced and a thorough vitrectomy is done. Triamcinolone can be used to stain the vitreous for easy visualization. Corneal tunnel is fashioned with a 2.8-mm keratome and a side port incision is framed midway between the left sclerotomy site and the corneal tunnel.

A three-piece foldable IOL is loaded and is injected into the eye. While doing so, the injector is withdrawn a bit in a way that the trailing haptic lies at the corneal incision. Glued IOL forceps are introduced from the left sclerotomy incision and the tip of the haptic is grasped followed by its externalization after the entire IOL has unfolded. The trailing haptic is flexed inside the eye and the "handshake technique"[21,22] is performed till the trailing haptic is externalized. Scleral pockets are made with a 26-gauge needle and the haptics are tucked. Vitrectomy is done at the sclerotomy site to cut down all the vitreous strands. Infusion is stopped, the scleral bed is dried, and glue is applied to seal the flaps. Fibrin glue can also be used to seal all the conjunctival peritomy sites and corneal incisions.

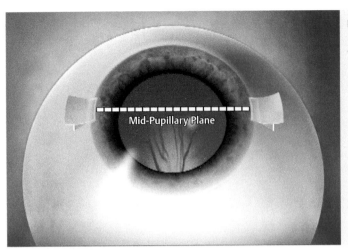

Fig. 15.12 Two partial-thickness flaps 180 degrees opposite to each other and the midpupillary plane axis.

15.8 No-Assistant Technique in Glued IOL

The no-assistant technique (NAT)[23] is a modified method of haptic externalization in glued IOL fixation technique of Agarwal et al. The technique derives its name from the fact that no assistant is needed to grab the leading haptic while the surgeon externalizes the trailing haptic. The leading haptic does not tend to slip back into the eye and lies continuously extruded throughout the procedure.

The technique works on the principle of "vector forces" and the midpupillary plane is a major contributor to the success of this technique (▶ Fig. 15.12). In the Agarwal method of glued IOL, the handshake technique[21] for trailing haptic is done below the midpupillary plane and the vector forces act in a way that the leading haptic tends to slip back into the eye, if not properly grasped by an assistant. The direction of vector forces change completely once the trailing haptic reaches or crosses the midpupillary plane (▶ Fig. 15.13). This causes further extrusion of the leading haptic from the sclerotomy site and abolishes the need for an assistant to hold the leading haptic. This phenomenon can be taken advantage of and many untoward incidents during the surgery can be avoided.

The initial steps of flap making, sclerotomy, and vitrectomy are the same as in a glued IOL surgery. A 23-gauge glued IOL forceps is introduced from the left sclerotomy site, the loaded cartridge is introduced into the eye, and the tip of the IOL haptic is grasped.

The IOL is slowly injected into the eye. Once the entire IOL has unfolded, the tip of the leading haptic is pulled and externalized. The surgeon flexes the trailing haptic with the glued IOL forceps in the right hand and introduces it into the eye so as to cross the midpupillary plane and reach more toward the 6 o'clock position. The surgeon now leaves the leading haptic and reintroduces the glued IOL forceps in the left hand from the side port incision into the eye.

The haptic is then transferred from the right glued IOL forceps to the left hand (handshake technique). The surgeon withdraws the right glued IOL forceps from the eye and reintroduces it from the right sclerotomy site. The trailing haptic is now transferred from the left hand to the right hand (handshake technique). The surgeon holds the haptic from its tip and externalizes by pulling it.

Scleral pocket is created with a 26-gauge needle parallel to the sclerotomy site along the edge of the flap. The haptics are tucked and vitrectomy is done to cut down any vitreous strands at the sclerotomy site. Fibrin glue is applied and the flaps are sealed along with all the conjunctival incisions. This technique is an attempt to make the process of haptic externalization, considered the most technically demanding part of the surgery, more easy and feasible.

15.9 Triumvirate Technique

This technique is a combination of modified PAL with IOL scaffold and glued IOL (▶ Fig. 15.14, ▶ Fig. 15.15, ▶ Fig. 15.16) in cases with PCR that have inadequate

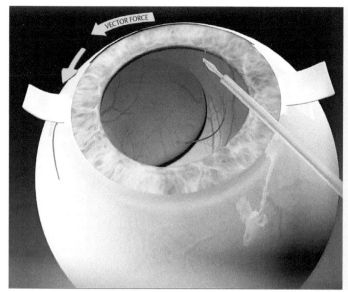

Fig. 15.13 Flexion of the trailing haptic beyond the midpupillary plane toward the 6 o'clock position. This reverses the direction of vector forces that lead to further exteriorization of the leading haptic and avoids the need for an assistant to grab the haptic to prevent it from slipping into the anterior chamber during the process of haptic externalization.

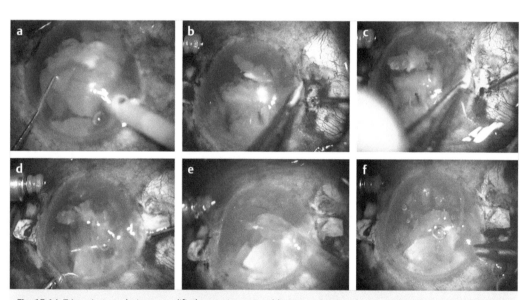

Fig. 15.14 Triumvirate technique: modified posterior assisted levitation (PAL) with intraocular lens (IOL) scaffold with glued IOL. **(a)** A posterior capsule rupture is noted during a phacoemulsification procedure. **(b)** Two partial-thickness scleral flaps are made 180 degrees opposite to each other as in glued IOL surgery. Sclerotomy is done with a 22-gauge needle 1 mm away from the limbus beneath the scleral flaps. **(c)** A rod is being inserted through the sclerotomy site. **(d)** The nuclear fragments are levitated into the anterior chamber (AC) with modified PAL technique. **(e)** A three-piece foldable IOL is injected beneath the nuclear fragments. **(f)** The IOL rests on the anterior surface of the iris tissue with nuclear pieces in the AC.

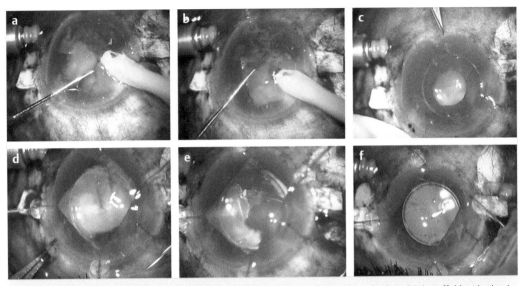

Fig. 15.15 Triumvirate technique: modified posterior assisted levitation with intraocular lens (IOL) scaffold with glued IOL. (a) Emulsification of the nuclear pieces being performed. (b) All the nuclear pieces are emulsified. (c) Corneal suture taken, IOL in the anterior chamber with cortical matter seen lying in the pupillary area. (d) Iris hooks are applied to enhance visualization. (e) Vitrectomy probe passed through the sclerotomy site and the cortical matter is cleaned up. (f) Entire cortical matter is cleaned.

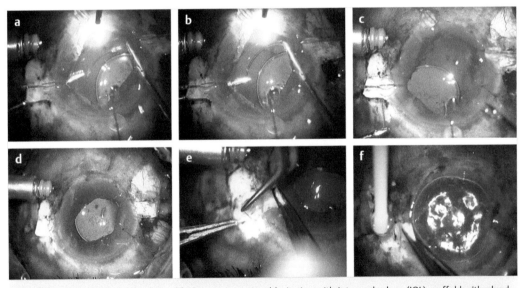

Fig. 15.16 Triumvirate technique: modified posterior assisted levitation with intraocular lens (IOL) scaffold with glued IOL. (a) Glued IOL forceps are introduced from the left sclerotomy site and the leading haptic is held with another glued IOL end-opening forceps. (b) The tip of the haptic is grasped to facilitate externalization. (c) The leading haptic is pulled and externalized. (d) Both haptics externalized. (e) The haptics are tucked into the scleral pockets. (f) Fibrin glue is applied beneath the scleral flaps.

capsular support and sinking nucleus with residual nuclear remnants to be emulsified.[25]

Following a PCR, two partial-thickness scleral flaps are made as in a glued IOL surgery followed by sclerotomy. A rod is inserted from the sclerotomy and placing the rod posterior to the nuclear fragment retrieves the sinking nucleus. A second rod can also be passed from the opposite sclerotomy site that is created for the glued IOL procedure. Passage of two rods from opposite direction enables and facilitates the nucleus retrieval into the AC. Once the nucleus is brought into AC, a three-piece foldable IOL is inserted beneath the nuclear fragments and the haptics of the IOL are made to rest on the anterior surface of the iris tissue (▶ Fig. 15.14). Phacoemulsification probe is introduced into the AC and the nucleus is emulsified. Phaco is done at low to moderate settings and the fragments are fed into the port of phaco probe in order to prevent any slippage of the fragments into the vitreous cavity from around the edges of the IOL (▶ Fig. 15.15).

The haptic of the IOL is then grasped with an end-opening glued IOL forceps and the handshake technique is done till the tip of the haptic is grasped. The haptics are then pulled from the tip and externalized (▶ Fig. 15.16). The haptics are tucked into the scleral pockets created with a 26-gauge needle and vitrectomy is performed at the sclerotomy site. Fibrin glue is applied beneath the scleral flaps and the conjunctival incisions are sealed.

In cases with dropped nucleus, triumvirate comprises sleeveless phacotip assisted levitation (SPAL)[26] with IOL scaffold and glued IOL. In SPAL, the sleeveless phacotip is passed from pars plana sclerotomy and the nucleus is lifted from the surface of the retina by vacuum from the tip of the phaco probe. Once the nucleus is levitated and is in midvitreous cavity, a short burst of phaco is applied, leading to embedment of phaco probe into the nucleus. The nucleus is then brought into the pupillary area and is lifted and placed onto the surface of iris. A three-piece foldable IOL is then injected beneath it as in an IOL scaffold procedure followed by glued fixation of the IOL.

15.10 Glued Intraocular Lens Scaffold

Glued IOL scaffold technique[27,28] is a combination of two previously described techniques of IOL scaffold and glued IOL. This technique is performed in cases of PCR with nonemulsified nuclear fragments with inadequate sulcus and iris support.

Following a PCR, the nuclear fragments are levitated into the AC and two partial-thickness scleral flaps are made 180 degrees opposite to each other. Sclerotomy is made with a 22-gauge needle about 1 to 1.5 mm away from the limbus. Fluid infusion is introduced into the eye and vitrectomy is performed with the vitrector introduced from the sclerotomy site. A three-piece foldable IOL is introduced into the AC beneath the nuclear fragments and the tip of the leading haptic is held with the glued IOL forceps introduced from the left sclerotomy site. The haptic is pulled and externalized, followed by externalization of the trailing haptic as in a glued IOL surgery. The variation in performing the glued IOL procedure initially here is that often the surgeon has to perform the procedure with the help of tactile sensations as the visualization of the haptic is often hampered due to the presence of nuclei in the AC. After the haptics have been tucked into the scleral pockets, an IOL scaffold procedure is performed. A phaco probe is introduced and all the nuclear fragments are emulsified with low to moderate settings.

The only limitation of this technique is that the surgeon should be well versed with both the glued IOL and IOL scaffold procedures.

15.11 Special Cases

15.11.1 Glued IOL Scaffold for Soemmering's Ring with PCR

The proliferation of the residual lens fibers along with the peripheral anterior and posterior capsular adhesions in long-standing cases of PCR often leads to the formation of Soemmering's ring (SR). These adhesions prevent the exposure of lens fibers to the aqueous and the surrounding environment promoting uninhibited growth of lens fibers. SR formation is often seen in pediatric cases that have undergone cataract surgery in early childhood. Glued IOL scaffold can be applied in these cases with feasible outcomes.[29]

As in a glued IOL procedure, a three-piece foldable IOL is injected in a way that the optic of the IOL lies beneath the SR material. Both the haptics are externalized and tucked into the scleral pockets (▶ Fig. 15.17). As SR has a typical peripheral disposition, iris hooks are often employed to enhance the visualization. The SR material is dislodged from the periphery into the center with the help of Sinskey's hook. Once dislodged, the iris hooks are removed and the SR material is emulsified with the phaco probe (▶ Fig. 15.18). Removal

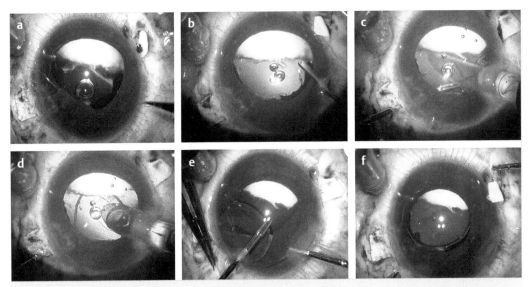

Fig. 15.17 Glued intraocular lens (IOL) scaffold for Soemmering's ring (SR) with posterior capsule rupture (PCR). **(a)** SR present along with PCR. Two scleral flaps made for glued IOL surgery. **(b)** Vitrectomy is done to clean up all the fibrotic membranous material around the SR. **(c)** A three-piece foldable IOL is introduced into the anterior chamber and the tip of the haptic grasped with glued IOL forceps introduced from the left sclerotomy site. **(d)** The IOL is injected and is slowly unfolded inside the eye. **(e)** The leading haptic is pulled and externalized and the trailing haptic is flexed inside the eye. **(f)** Both haptics externalized with the optic lying beneath the SR material.

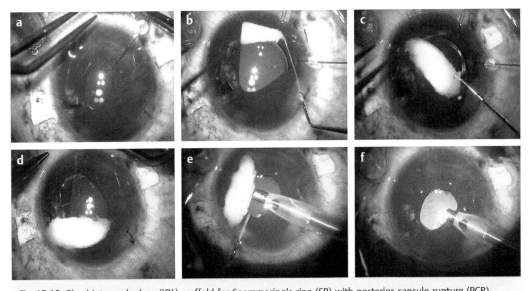

Fig. 15.18 Glued intraocular lens (IOL) scaffold for Soemmering's ring (SR) with posterior capsule rupture (PCR). **(a)** Both the haptics are tucked into scleral pockets. Iris hooks are placed to enhance the visualization of SR. **(b)** SR is then displaced centrally with Sinskey's hook. **(c)** The SR lying above the IOL optic. **(d)** Iris hooks are removed to prevent the slippage of SR from around the edges of the IOL optic. **(e)** The SR material is emulsified with phacoemulsification probe. **(f)** A well-placed IOL with SR removal seen at the end of procedure.

of the iris hooks prevents the slippage of SR material from around the edges of the optic of IOL into the vitreous cavity. Stromal hydration is done and the corneal wound is sutured with a 10–0 nylon. Fibrin glue is applied and the scleral flaps are sealed.

15.11.2 Glued IOL Scaffold for Traumatic Subluxated Lens

In the cases with massively subluxated lens, the glued IOL scaffold procedure can be performed where initially vitrectomy is performed beneath the subluxated lens to cut down all the vitreous adhesions surrounding the lens and its trimming if present in the AC.[27]

In these cases, the optic of the three-piece IOL is positioned beneath the lens nucleus and the glued IOL scaffold procedure is performed. While the IOL is being inserted, a rod passed from the opposite sclerotomy site can support the nucleus from behind and prevent it from dropping into the vitreous cavity. The lens is then emulsified with a phaco probe as in a glued IOL scaffold procedure (▶ Fig. 15.19, ▶ Fig. 15.20).

15.11.3 Pupil Expansion Devices in Posterior Capsular Rupture

Inadequate pupil dilation is often encountered intraoperatively during a PCR. The most important aspect at this stage is to understand and know the kind of pupil expansion device (PED) that works best for the surgical case. Intraocular devices such as pupil expansion rings should be avoided, as there are chances of the ring getting dislodged into the vitreous cavity. Under such circumstances, the surgeon should use iris hooks that is a kind of externally fixated device with virtually no chance of getting dislodged into the posterior segment. Iris hooks are the most commonly employed PED, but the disadvantage with iris hooks is that it needs separate additional side port incisions to be framed and while employing hooks, care should be taken that the hooks do not catch the capsulorhexis margin or engage the anterior capsule tears as it engages the pupil in the anteroposterior direction.

15.12 Complications

Complications are an inherent part of any surgery and the incidences of complications that can

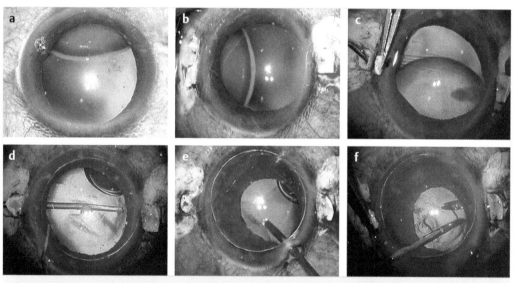

Fig. 15.19 Glued intraocular lens (IOL) scaffold for traumatic subluxated lens. **(a)** Eccentrically located traumatic subluxated lens. **(b)** With the surgeon seated temporally two partial-thickness scleral flaps made 180 degrees opposite to each other. **(c)** Sclerotomy made with 22-gauge needle about 1 mm away from the limbus beneath the scleral flaps. **(d)** Posterior assisted levitation done with a rod passed from the sclerotomy site. **(e)** Vitrectomy being performed beneath the lens to cut all vitreous strands. **(f)** A three-piece foldable IOL is injected below the lens and the haptics are externalized. The optic of the IOL acts as a scaffold.

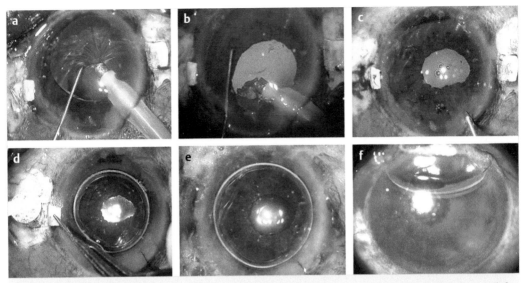

Fig. 15.20 Glued intraocular lens (IOL) scaffold for traumatic subluxated lens. **(a)** Phaco probe introduced to emulsify the nucleus lying in anterior chamber. **(b)** The nucleus is being emulsified. **(c)** The entire nucleus is emulsified. Corneal suture is taken and the wound is secured with a 10–0 nylon. **(d)** Fibrin glue is applied beneath the scleral flaps. **(e)** Both the scleral flaps and the conjunctival wounds are sealed with glue. **(f)** Postoperative image of the case.

lead to suboptimal outcomes following a PCR are enormous.

Intraoperatively, the most common complication of PCR can be a nucleus or a nuclear fragment drop. In the event of a rupture of the posterior lens capsule, the surgeon must avoid any uncontrolled and forceful surgical maneuvers in the vitreous cavity in an attempt to retrieve the sinking lens fragments. Any retrieval technique that does not provide for the appropriate management of the vitreous first creates the potential of immediate or subsequent retinal complications. Small lens fragments consisting of mostly cortical material may gradually resolve with conservative medical management alone. However, large lens fragments with a sizable nuclear component do not resolve easily, and may elicit a phaco antigenic response from the host. Hence, it is extremely essential to remove the larger chunks of nuclear fragments from the vitreous cavity.

An IOL dislocation or a drop can also occur either intraoperatively or in the postoperative period. Cystoids macular edema is often seen following a vitreous disturbance and in extreme cases of vitreous traction, retinal detachment has also been reported. The posterior segment complications should invite for a prompt referral of the patient to a vitreoretinal surgeon.

15.13 Discussion

Retinal detachment, cystoid macular edema, uveitis, and glaucoma are associated with the complication of PCR with vitreous loss in cataract extraction. Expedited referral to vitreoretinal specialists is recommended for management of posterior segment complications following a PC break. A careful anterior vitrectomy should be performed to minimize the vitreous disturbance and prevent further complications. Preoperative risk factors such as miosis, restlessness, zonulopathy, and floppy iris syndrome should be taken into consideration and the surgical plan should be charted accordingly with all the contingency plans ready. Restless patients may be managed with appropriate sedation and anesthesia. A careful and systematic approach in patients may have good outcomes in the setting of PCR. Recent advancements in techniques have led to new standards of care and management and help optimize the results in complicated cases.

15.14 Key Pearls

- Subsequent to an intraoperative PCR, the AC should be stabilized with an OVD injected from the side port incision followed by withdrawal of the phaco probe.

- Adequate vitrectomy should be performed preferably from the pars plana site as it allows retropupillary access to the vitreous and prevents further prolapse of vitreous into the AC.
- In the case of miosis, iris hooks should be employed for peripheral visualization of the cortex and to assess other intraoperative details.
- IOL scaffold technique helps emulsify the nonemulsified nuclear fragments in the presence of a PCR.
- PAL and modified PAL help levitate the nuclear fragments from the anterior vitreous into the AC.
- Modified PAL has an added advantage that the sclerotomy site gets covered by the scleral flap and hence there is no need to suture the site. Moreover, when glued IOL is being performed, two sites are available from where the modified PAL can be performed. This allows better control and levitation of the nucleus into the AC.

Videos

Video 15.1 Sulcus placement of an intraocular lens (IOL) in posterior capsule rupture. Intraoperative posterior capsule rupture is observed and iris hooks are placed to enhance the visualization. Fluid infusion is introduced inside the eye and anterior vitrectomy is performed with the removal of peripheral cortex. A three-piece IOL is eventually placed in the sulcus.

Video 15.2 Posterior assisted levitation and intraocular lens (IOL) scaffold. The sinking nucleus is retrieved into the anterior chamber with posterior assisted levitation method through the pars plana site. The nucleus is brought into the anterior chamber and three-piece IOL is inserted beneath the fragments and an IOL scaffold is performed. The IOL is securely placed in the sulcus above the capsulorhexis margin.

Video 15.3 Sleeveless phacotip assisted levitation (SPAL) with intraocular lens (IOL) scaffold. The dropped nucleus is levitated with SPAL technique into the anterior chamber and an IOL scaffold is performed. The three-piece IOL is then dialed into the sulcus.

Video 15.4 Refractive glued intraocular lens (IOL) exchange. Refractive error of 7 diopters was noted on the second postoperative day. Therefore, the IOL was explanted by lifting the scleral flaps and a new three-piece IOL with correct refractive power was inserted inside the eye.

Video 15.5 Triumvirate technique. The video demonstrates the technique of triumvirate that

comprises modified posterior assisted levitation with intraocular lens (IOL) scaffold and glued IOL procedure in cases with deficient sulcus support and sinking nucleus.

Video 15.6 Glued intraocular lens (IOL) scaffold. This video encompasses all the details of glued IOL scaffold procedure along with the technique and associated difficulties. (This video is provided courtesy of Amar Agarwal.)

Video 15.7 Gluing the intraocular lens (IOL) beneath the subluxated cataractous lens. This video demonstrates the applicability of glued IOL scaffold procedure for subluxated lenses.

Video 15.8 Glued intraocular lens (IOL) scaffold for Soemmering's ring. In aphakic cases, the glued IOL procedure is performed initially followed by dislodgement of Soemmering's ring from the periphery into the center of the optic of the IOL. The Soemmering material is then emulsified with a phaco probe. (This video is provided courtesy of Amar Agarwal.)

Video 15.9 Phimotic capsular bag–intraocular lens (IOL) complex dislocation. The fibrotic bag–IOL complex is explanted and a new three-piece IOL is fixated with glued IOL technique.

Video 15.10 L-shaped scleral incision with refractive intraocular lens (IOL) exchange with Soemmering's ring and glued IOL. The video demonstrates the case of a young girl with pseudophakia who had a refractive error of 7 diopters and prolapsed IOL in anterior chamber with 270-degree iridocapsular adhesions, a Soemmering ring, and a posterior capsular yttrium aluminum garnet opening.

Video 15.11 No-assistant technique for glued intraocular lens (IOL). The no-assistant technique is a method of haptic externalization employed for glued IOL procedure that does not need an assistant to hold the leading haptic from slipping inside the eye.

Video 15.12 Handshake technique for glued intraocular lens. The video demonstrates handshake technique for haptic externalization that involves the transfer of haptics from one hand to another till the tip of the haptic is grasped and is externalized. (This video is provided courtesy of Amar Agarwal.)

Video 15.13 Complications of glued intraocular lens (IOL). This video showcases all the complications that can occur in a glued IOL surgery. (This video is provided courtesy of Amar Agarwal.)

References

[1] Asaria RHY, Wong SC, Sullivan PM. Risk for posterior capsule rupture after vitreoretinal surgery. J Cataract Refract Surg. 2006; 32(6):1068–1069

[2] Novak MA, Rice TA, Michels RG, Auer C. The crystalline lens after vitrectomy for diabetic retinopathy. Ophthalmology. 1984; 91(12):1480–1484

[3] Faulborn J, Conway BP, Machemer R. Surgical complications of pars plana vitreous surgery. Ophthalmology. 1978; 85(2): 116–125

[4] Gimbel HV. Posterior capsule tears using phacoemulsification causes, prevention and management. Eur J Implant Refract Surg.. 1990; 2:63–69

[5] Arbisser LB, Charles S, Howcroft M, Werner L. Management of vitreous loss and dropped nucleus during cataract surgery. Ophthalmol Clin North Am. 2006; 19(4):495–506

[6] Angunawela RI, Liyanage SE, Wong SC, Little BC. Intraocular pressure and visual outcomes following intracameral triamcinolone assisted anterior vitrectomy in complicated cataract surgery. Br J Ophthalmol. 2009; 93(12):1691–1692

[7] Fine HF, Spaide RF. Visualization of the posterior precortical vitreous pocket in vivo with triamcinolone. Arch Ophthalmol. 2006; 124(11):1663

[8] Gillies MC, Simpson JM, Billson FA, et al. Safety of an intravitreal injection of triamcinolone: results from a randomized clinical trial. Arch Ophthalmol. 2004; 122(3):336–340

[9] Burk SE, Da Mata AP, Snyder ME, Schneider S, Osher RH, Cionni RJ. Visualizing vitreous using Kenalog suspension. J Cataract Refract Surg. 2003; 29(4):645–651

[10] Kasbekar S, Prasad S, Kumar BV. Clinical outcomes of triamcinolone-assisted anterior vitrectomy after phacoemulsification complicated by posterior capsule rupture. J Cataract Refract Surg. 2013; 39(3):414–418

[11] Peyman GA, Cheema R, Conway MD, Fang T. Triamcinolone acetonide as an aid to visualization of the vitreous and the posterior hyaloid during pars plana vitrectomy. Retina. 2000; 20(5):554–555

[12] Enaida H, Hata Y, Ueno A, et al. Possible benefits of triamcinolone-assisted pars plana vitrectomy for retinal diseases. Retina. 2003; 23(6):764–770

[13] Packard RBS, Kinnear FC. Manual of Cataract and Intraocular Lens Surgery. Edinburgh: Churchill Livingstone; 1991:47

[14] Kelman C.. Posterior capsular rupture: technique PAL. Video J Cataract Refract Surg. 1996; 12:30

[15] Kelman CD. Posterior assisted levitation. In: Burrato L, ed. Phacoemulsification: principles and techniques. Thorofare, NJ: Slack Incorporated; 1998:511–512

[16] Chang DF, Packard RB. Posterior assisted levitation for nucleus retrieval using Viscoat after posterior capsule rupture. J Cataract Refract Surg. 2003; 29(10):1860–1865

[17] Kumar DA, Agarwal A, Prakash G, Jacob S, Agarwal A, Sivagnanam S. IOL scaffold technique for posterior capsule rupture. J Refract Surg. 2012; 28(5):314–315

[18] Narang P, Agarwal A, Kumar DA, Jacob S, Agarwal A, Agarwal A. Clinical outcomes of intraocular lens scaffold surgery: a one-year study. Ophthalmology. 2013; 120 (12):2442–2448

[19] Gimbel HV, DeBroff BM. Intraocular lens optic capture. J Cataract Refract Surg. 2004; 30(1):200–206

[20] Agarwal A, Kumar DA, Jacob S, Baid C, Agarwal A, Srinivasan S. Fibrin glue-assisted sutureless posterior chamber intraocular lens implantation in eyes with deficient posterior capsules. J Cataract Refract Surg. 2008; 34(9):1433–1438

[21] Agarwal A, Jacob S, Kumar DA, Narasimhan S, Agarwal A. Handshake technique for glued intrascleral haptic fixation of a posterior chamber intraocular lens. J Cataract Refract Surg. 2013; 39(3):317–322

[22] Narang P, Agarwal A. The "correct shake" for "handshake" in glued intrascleral fixation of intraocular lens. Indian J Ophthalmol. 2016; 64(11):854–856

[23] Narang P. Modified method of haptic externalization of posterior chamber intraocular lens in fibrin glue-assisted intrascleral fixation: no-assistant technique. J Cataract Refract Surg. 2013; 39(1):4–7

[24] Agarwal A, Narang P, Kumar DA, Agarwal A. Trocar anterior chamber maintainer: improvised infusion technique. J Cataract Refract Surg. 2016; 42(2):185–189

[25] Narang P, Agarwal A. Modified posterior-assisted levitation with intraocular lens scaffold and glued IOL for sinking nucleus in eyes with inadequate sulcus support. J Cataract Refract Surg. 2017; 43(7):872–876

[26] Agarwal A, Narang P, A Kumar D, Agarwal A. Clinical outcomes of sleeveless phacotip assisted levitation of dropped nucleus. Br J Ophthalmol. 2014; 98(10):1429–1434

[27] Agarwal A, Jacob S, Agarwal A, Narasimhan S, Kumar DA, Agarwal A. Glued intraocular lens scaffolding to create an artificial posterior capsule for nucleus removal in eyes with posterior capsule tear and insufficient iris and sulcus support. J Cataract Refract Surg. 2013; 39(3):326–333

[28] Narang P, Agarwal A, Kumar DA, Agarwal A. Clinical outcomes of the glued intraocular lens scaffold. J Cataract Refract Surg. 2015; 41(9):1867–1874

[29] Narang P, Agarwal A, Kumar DA. Glued intraocular lens scaffolding for Soemmerring ring removal in aphakia with posterior capsule defect. J Cataract Refract Surg. 2015; 41(4): 708–713

Part IV

Miscellaneous

16 MiLoop: Micro-Interventional, Phaco-Free, Lens Fragmentation

Tsontcho Ianchulev and Susan MacDonald

Abstract

The chapter describes a new device "miLoop" that is a micro-interventional device for cataract surgery that helps divide the nucleus with the "loop," thereby reducing the phaco energy that is employed in cataract surgery and also has an added advantage of reducing the size of incision in a small-incision cataract surgery.

Keywords: miLoop, lens fragmentation, zero phaco lensectomy, endocapsular fragmentation

16.1 Rationale and Background

Dr. Kelman introduced phacoemulsification around 50 years ago and in the developed world it is currently the standard mode to perform cataract surgery. In the United States, more than 3.5 million cataract surgeries are performed every year, of which more than 95% are done with standard phacoemulsification. Incremental advances in phacoemulsification have led to minimally invasive, highly efficient, and safe cataract surgery with small clear corneal incisions (< 2.8 mm) that transmit reduced ultrasound energy to the eye (e.g., torsional phaco) with relatively few complications. More than 95% of eyes achieve better than 20/40 best-corrected visual acuity (BCVA) postoperatively. Nevertheless, the conventional phacoemulsification paradigm has plateaued on the innovation curve, and incremental changes have not been able to solve for the ever-increasing demands of both surgeons and patients. Patients undergo cataract surgery much earlier on the disease spectrum, often with very early cataracts (sometimes even clear lens extraction with BCVA 20/20), many well before the end of their life expectancy with 20% having cataract surgery before the age of 60 years[1] with more than 20 years of their lifespan remaining.

This is redefining the risk–benefit equation of cataract surgery, raising the safety bar to the level of refractive procedures such as laser in situ keratomileusis (LASIK). Yet, phacoemulsification continues to deliver significant amounts of heat-generating, burst energy to the eye (▶ Fig. 16.1, ▶ Fig. 16.2), which can permanently destroy more than 10 to 15% of the corneal endothelium—a fragile and important cellular layer of corneal tissue that does not regenerate and continues to undergo atrophic aging changes throughout life with 1 to 2% reduction per year. With more advanced cataracts, the changes are more prominent and endothelial cell loss can exceed 40%. Even with best-in-class equipment and surgical technique, patients continue to experience phaco-related complications such as capsular tear, corneal edema, iritis, and endothelial cell loss.

In the developing world, phacoemulsification has had a slow adoption. This is due to several factors, including the expense of the technology and disposables, the maintenance of the equipment and the steep, long learning curve of the surgical technique. The maturity and density of the cataracts make them technically difficult and require a

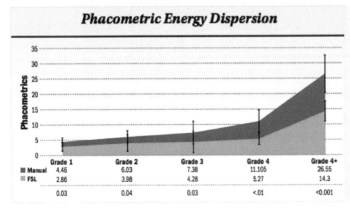

Phacometric Energy Dispersion

	Grade 1	Grade 2	Grade 3	Grade 4	Grade 4+
■ Manual	4.46	6.03	7.38	11.105	26.55
■ FSL	2.86	3.98	4.28	5.27	14.3
	0.03	0.04	0.03	<.01	<0.001

Fig. 16.1 Increasing levels of phaco energy used with higher grade cataracts.

ALL CURRENT TECHNIQUES

1. Rely on potential fracture plane creation and propagation

2. Use two instrument fracture

3. Use centrifugal, side-ways separation with capsule stress

4. Prone to Inconsistent nuclear disassembly; not surefire

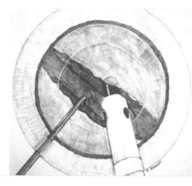

Fig. 16.2 Demonstration of the current technique and principles of phacoemulsification. Conventional phaco chopping techniques are centrifugal (in–out) with significant tension on the capsular complex.

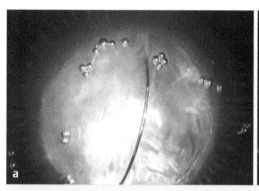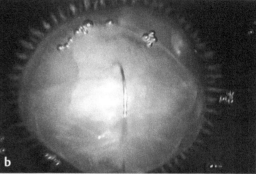

Fig. 16.3 (a,b) Miyake's view of miLoop full-thickness endocapsular nucleus disassembly, demonstrating minimal stress of the capsular bag zonules.

substantial amount of phaco-ultrasound energy. In fact, there are many who believe small-incision cataract surgery (SICS) is a superior surgical choice for these cases, because dense cataracts are challenging even for the expert phaco surgeon and may be best served by extracapsular and manual small-incision cataract surgery (MSICS or SICS) techniques. In fact, a randomized control trial demonstrated SICS to be economical[2] and nearly as effective as phacoemulsification.[3,4]There is a difference of 0.3 to 0.5 diopter of astigmatism between SICS and phaco, but most significant was the substantial difference in cost. A version of SICS is being taught and popularized the world over by major international nongovernmental developmental organizations. SICS does reduce an extracapsular cataract incision size, to 7-mm external incision with a 9-mm internal width. This "small-incision" extracapsular is still a large incision (7 mm); many times, it may need to be sutured and/or may widen to safely remove the natural lens.

Recently, the first micro-interventional device for cataract surgery, the miLoop, was developed and introduced by Dr. Ianchulev at the American Society

of Cataract and Refractive Surgery (ASCRS) meeting (Los Angeles, 2017). Using first-in-class Nitinol technology, the miLoop is following the recent advent of micro-stents and minimally invasive glaucoma surgery (MIGS) technology, which are already changing the treatment paradigm for glaucoma (e.g., iStent, CyPass). This device has been used to reduce phaco energy in cataracts and recently has been used to reduce the size of SICS incision.

16.2 MiLoop Device

The miLoop is a super-elastic nitinol microthin filament around 300 μm in diameter. It can be introduced through a 1.5-mm incision and is designed for endocapsular deployment without exerting tension on the posterior capsule. In expanded position, it achieves a memory-shaped loop that encircles the lens and upon contraction creates full-thickness nuclear cuts that can be repeated for end-to-end cataract segmentation (▶ Fig. 16.3). When used as an adjunct to phacoemulsification (i.e., mi-phaco technique), it can facilitate the lens breakup and removal and minimize the need for phaco energy.

This microthin nitinol filament allows the surgeon to do lens fragmentation with a new micro-interventional technique without using the phaco probe and without using a second instrument.

Conventional chopping or prechopping techniques that use centrifugal (in–out) forces are of variable effectiveness depending on the hardness of the lens nucleus.

It is a two-instrument technique that uses phaco energy to cleave the nucleus and is variable in achieving full-thickness reliable fragmentation because it relies on the propagation of a fragmentation cleavage plane (▶ Fig. 16.4) through the lenticular complex from a surface chop, which is highly dependent on the density and compliance of the nucleus. It is also invariably centrifugal in nature with out–in cleavage forces that can destabilize and exert tension on the capsular complex.

MiLoop's endocapsular full-thickness lens fragmentation has several advantages. It allows nuclear disassembly of cataracts independent of cataract grade, utilizing out–in, centripetal cutting rather than centrifugal forces (▶ Fig. 16.5). The technique reduces stress on the zonules and reduces the risk of zonular dehiscence and capsular bag instability. It is a technique that is simple to learn and limits the stress on the capsular bag. It has been found to be a useful nuclear disassembly technique.

16.3 New Surgical Technique for Nucleus Disassembly

MiLoop fragmentation is unique and unconventional in its mechanistic approach to the nucleus. For the first time, it allows the ability to achieve zero-energy, centripetal (out–in) nucleus disassembly that is materially different from all conventional techniques of in–out, centrifugal chopping and fragmentation (▶ Fig. 16.5). It completes full-thickness microsegmentation and disassembly regardless of cataract grade through a single 1.5-mm incision. It also allows fragmentation to occur under viscoelastic control without phaco probe in the eye and

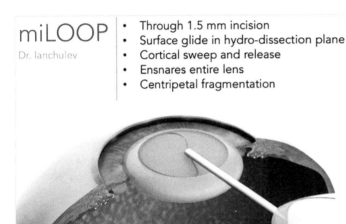

miLOOP

Dr. Ianchulev

- Through 1.5 mm incision
- Surface glide in hydro-dissection plane
- Cortical sweep and release
- Ensnares entire lens
- Centripetal fragmentation

Fig. 16.4 MiLoop expansion in the horizontal hydrodissection plane prior to endocapsular rotation.

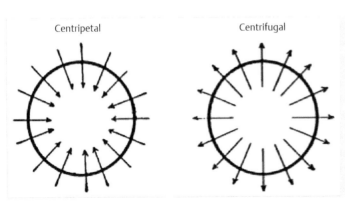

Centripetal   Centrifugal

Fig. 16.5 Centripetal (out–in) versus centrifugal forces (in–out). Outward force vectors exert more stretch pressure on the capsular bag.

any irrigation and aspiration, further protecting the endothelium from phacoemulsification-related exposure during the disassembly step of surgery.

16.3.1 Clinical Application

The miLoop enables a highly versatile surgical approach that can be applied across the spectrum of cataract intervention. It can be used as a stand-alone as well as an adjunct to phacoemulsification. As a very new technology and a completely different method of nucleus disassembly, its clinical applications are yet to be fully understood and explored.

Initial experiences by Drs. Lanchulev and MacDonald have found high utility in advanced cataracts (grade 3 +) as well as in cases of capsular instability (pseudoexfoliation) and small pupils. It is also useful in any case where reducing phaco-burst energy exposure is important (weak endothelium, younger patients).

16.4 Description of Technique

After the completion of capsulotomy, the instrument tip is introduced through a clear cornea incision into the anterior chamber filled with ophthalmic viscosurgical device (OVD). Advancing a sliding actuation button on the handle opens the nitinol filament within the capsular bag. The initial expansion of the loop is performed in the coronal plane just beneath the anterior capsule (▶ Fig. 16.3). The surgeon next sweeps the fully expanded loop back along the hydrodissection plane against the internal capsular contour until it encircles the nucleus in the sagittal plane. Sliding the hand piece button backward contracts the loop until it has completely transected the nucleus. For denser nuclei, a second instrument may be used to steady the nucleus as it is being cut. After rotating the nucleus, the same maneuvers are repeated to divide the nucleus into quadrants. An additional optional cut to divide the nucleus into six pieces can be performed.

From the existing experience, one can classify its main applications into three categories:

- MiLoop with I/A for grade 1 and 2 cataracts (Zero-Phaco Lensectomy). In the cases of soft cataract, the miLoop can easily disassemble the nuclear complex, which can then be evacuated with aspiration without any phaco power—as clearly demonstrated by Dr. Bill Wiley (ASCRS 2017). The miLoop endocapsular fragmentation

in addition with the miLoop cortical microdissection and release from the peripheral sweep enables fast and efficient, phaco-free surgery with no burst energy exposure to the endothelium—which is a significant advantage for premium IOL cases, clear lens extractions, as well as surgery in young patients.

- MiLoop with phaco for grade 3 and 4 + cataracts (miPHACO) for reduced energy and tissue damage. A randomized controlled study presented at the ASCRS 2016 meeting (Ianchulev, MacDonald, Koo, Chang), in press at the time of this publication, demonstrated significant improvement in phaco efficiency with 40% reduction over phaco alone in the hands of highly experienced phaco surgeons using the most advanced phaco torsional equipment by Alcon. There was improvement in energy and fluidics as well as safety of standard phaco with adjunct nucleus disassembly with the miLoop.

- MiLoop miniCAP for any grade cataract (miniCAP): from SICS to minimally invasive manual cataract surgery through 4-mm scleral pocket. This technique was first described by MacDonald and Ianchulev. After a paracentesis incision is placed, the anterior capsule is stained with trypan blue. A 4-mm scleral incision is made 2 mm posterior to the limbus and is carried forward into 1 mm of clear cornea that is then flared out on each side of the pocket, expanding the pocket up to a total of 6 mm. Once the pocket is created, the wound is opened into the anterior chamber and a continuous curvilinear capsulorhexis or can-opener capsulorrhexis is performed. After hydrodissection, the miLoop is used to divide the nucleus into four pieces. As the miLoop is dividing the nucleus, the second pass is used to bring the nucleus into the anterior chamber. An irrigating lens loop is then used to gently remove the individual fragments.

16.5 Clinical Study

This was a prospective, multisurgeon, randomized controlled trial performed at the Ophthalmic Surgical Center, Panama. One eye from each of 100 subjects was randomized to either conventional phacoemulsification or phacoemulsification preceded by adjunct micro-interventional nuclear fragmentation with miLoop. There was a 20% higher endothelial cell loss trend in the phaco-only group.

This study is the first clinical comparison of micro-interventional miLoop-assisted phacoemulsification to standard phacoemulsification. In an effort to test the efficacy and safety of miLoop, a population comprised exclusively of advanced cataracts was selected. As an adjunctive method of presegmenting the nucleus, the miLoop technique was 100% effective in fragmenting every dense nucleus within the capsular bag. There were no instances of zonular dialysis or anterior or posterior capsule tears occurring during miLoop nuclear segmentation.

16.6 Discussion

MiLoop is a promising new technology that has been shown to reduce endothelial cell loss when combined with phacoemulsification techniques. It is showing great promise in the developing world, improving the SICS technique and introducing small incision of less than 3.5 to 4 mm, creating the minicamp, a new technique that has the potential to revolutionize nonphacoemulsification in developing countries.

16.7 Key Pearls

- MiLoop allows endocapsular fragmentation of nucleus with the help of a "loop" that is

introduced inside the capsular bag, followed by engulfment of the entire nucleus and then cutting it across by withdrawal of the loop.
- In soft cataracts, miLoop disassembles the nuclear complex easily and in cases of grade 3 to 4 cataracts, it reduces the use of effective phaco energy by 40%.
- MiLoop reduces the size of SICS as it reduces the effective size of nucleus that is to be removed from the eye.

References

[1] DeBry P, Olson RJ, Crandall AS. Comparison of energy required for phaco-chop and divide and conquer phacoemulsification. J Cataract Refract Surg. 1998; 24(5):689–692

[2] Ram J, Wesendahl TA, Auffarth GU, Apple DJ. Evaluation of in situ fracture versus phaco chop techniques. J Cataract Refract Surg. 1998; 24(11):1464–1468

[3] Wong T, Hingorani M, Lee V. Phacoemulsification time and power requirements in phaco chop and divide and conquer nucleofractis techniques. J Cataract Refract Surg. 2000; 26(9): 1374–1378

[4] Pirazzoli G, D'Eliseo D, Ziosi M, Acciarri R. Effects of phacoemulsification time on the corneal endothelium using phacofracture and phaco chop techniques. J Cataract Refract Surg. 1996; 22(7):967–969

17 Keratoconus and Cataract Surgery

Arthur B. Cummings and Sheraz Daya

Abstract

Irregular astigmatism associated with keratoconus usually leads to a dissatisfied patient with suboptimal outcomes postcataract surgery. This chapter expresses all the concerns and the guidelines to be followed to minimize the postsurgery refractive error and also highlights the intraocular lens (IOL) power calculations and the choice of IOL options that are available.

Keywords: keratoconus, hard contact lens, toric IOL, astigmatism, irregular astigmatism, corneal optics

17.1 Introduction

One of the greatest challenges in modern cataract surgery is that of getting the refractive target right. Patients want and expect good refractive outcomes from cataract surgery today. From the most basic surgical perspective, however, surgeons want to replace the cloudy crystalline lens with a pristine intraocular lens (IOL) that allows all light to pass through it. Keratoconus (and other conditions causing irregular corneal astigmatism) adds a level of complexity to this aspect. Not only is biometry a lot more challenging, but also, sometimes, despite the newly placed IOL being pristine and in the correct position and alignment, the best-corrected acuity does not improve as much as what was expected. In eyes with keratoconus and cataract, both the irregular corneal optics and the cloudy lens optics are playing a role in the reduced vision. To manage patient expectations best, it is prudent to know what the cornea's contribution is to the reduced vision before embarking on the cataract surgery.

Just like cataracts, keratoconic corneas also come is varying grades of distortion. For this chapter, perhaps the Amsler–Krumeich classification will work best to grade corneal irregularity. Preoperative vision, both UDVA (uncorrected distance visual acuity) and BSCVA (best spectacle corrected visual acuity) as well as the visual history some years prior to cataract surgery are also very helpful. For most cataract patients, the cause of the recent reduction in vision will be the cataracts as keratoconus tends to be more stable at ages at which cataracts typically occur. If the vision prior to the onset of cataracts could be well corrected

with spectacles to a level of 6/12 or better, then cataract surgery with or without toric implants should provide similar or better best-corrected spectacle vision. Good vision with soft contact lenses (CLs), including toric soft CLs, may well be a similar indicator; however, soft lenses can mask a level of irregularity that may be significant and best to seek out records of best spectacle corrected vision from the individual responsible for fitting the lens. If the patient requires rigid gas permeable CLs (RGPs) or scleral or mini-scleral CLs to see well, cataract surgery may provide disappointing visual results until the corneal irregularity is addressed. Of course, patients can continue to wear RGPs or scleral CLs following cataract surgery, but when patient expectations are considered, it is usually desirable to provide the best UDVA wherever possible. Today addressing corneal irregularities is more successful than years before with the use of topography-guided laser ablation and intracorneal ring segments (▶ Fig. 17.1) and if the cornea has

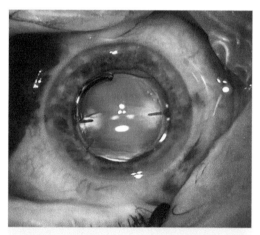

Fig. 17.1 Intraoperative image of a Bitoric lens implant in a patient with keratoconus following earlier implantation of a Ferrara ring. The patient was an elderly gas permeable contact lens wearer who historically had best spectacle corrected visual acuity (BSCVA) of 6/21 and became contact lens intolerant. A Ferrara ring was used to improve her corneal shape with improved BSCVA to 6/15. Microincisional cataract surgery was performed through a scleral incision and a 3.0-diopter Bitoric lens implant inserted. Postoperatively her uncorrected visual acuity improved to 6/12 and BSCVA to 6/9 with a refraction of + 1.25 − 1.00 × 160.

been regularized prior to cataract surgery, improved outcomes can be expected.

17.1.1 Other Grading Systems for Keratoconus

- Belin's ABCD classification[1]:
  - **A**nterior corneal curvature.
  - Posterior corneal curvature (**B**ack).
  - **C**orneal pachymetry.
  - Corrected distance visual acuity (CDVA; **D**istance vision, corrected).
- RETICS (Redes Temáticas de Investigación Cooperativa en Salud—Thematic Networks of Cooperative Research in Health). This classification is based mainly on CDVA but also includes higher-order aberrations (HOAs) like coma, asphericity, internal astigmatism, and H-RMS, thereby providing a functional classification of visual acuity. Using RETICS, toric IOLs can be implanted in eyes with grade 1 and selected eyes with grade 2. For higher grades, it makes sense to try and regularize the cornea first by means of intrastromal corneal ring segments (ISCRS) or topography-guided photorefractive keratectomy (TG-PRK).

17.1.2 Intraocular Lens Power Calculations in Keratoconus

IOL power calculations use corneal data in two ways:
- To apportion optical power as part of the entire optical system (e.g., 43 diopters). The cornea provides 66% of the refractive power of the eye, so even a 2% error can lead to a miscalculation of 1.00 diopters.
- As a predictor of where the IOL will land up within the eye (ELP or effective lens position). The effect of ELP can be summarized by this rule of thumb: a 1-mm shift in the anteroposterior position of the IOL causes a 10% change in the effective IOL power. An eye with a 23.00-diopter IOL that lands up 0.5 mm more anteriorly than predicted will be 1.15 diopters more myopic than expected.

In biometry, the cornea is characterized by the K-value, a single number that assigns refractive power to the cornea. Normally, this would suffice in regular corneas, but when the cornea is irregular and multifocal, a single number fails to provide sufficient data for biometry. Which part of the multifocal cornea is the patient using when looking in the distance? Is this the same part of the cornea when looking up close? Does this change during the day or during the visual task depending on fatigue, working distance and position, nature of the visual task, and so the list of variables goes on? What single K-value is going to be able to provide the best information for the IOL formulae? To add to the error for potential, consider how all keratometers work. They project an image onto the cornea and then measure the size of the reflected image. This size of the image is then converted to a measure of corneal steepness in millimeters of radius. A flatter cornea leads to a larger image and a steeper cornea to a smaller image. Given the mechanics, one can now clearly see how something as simple as misalignment may impact a corneal steepness measurement. The steepness or curvature is converted to a dioptric power using the formula $D = (i - 1)/r$, where i is the refractive index (RI) of the cornea and r is the radius of curvature in meters. This formula is an approximation as it ignores the posterior cornea curvature. A further error may creep in with the assumption that the RI of the cornea is 1.3375 for all humans. It is, however, highly likely that there is wide variation in the RI of the human cornea, both in its virgin state and following refractive surgery. It is likely to be different too in abnormal corneas such as we find in keratoconus. Because we cannot measure the corneal RI for any individual patient, we substitute with an assumption.

17.1.3 Biometry, Intraocular Lens Formulae, and Corneal Optics

The central corneal shape, the most important corneal power for most everyday tasks, is best described as an aspheric–toric surface. Aspheric because it is typically steeper in the center and flatter in the periphery and toric because most corneas have some degree of regular astigmatism, even if very subtle. Over and above these lower-order aberrations, there are also HOAs or irregularities. When these are amplified as with keratoconus, they can take on clinical and visual significance. These irregularities are usually described with Zernike polynomials or Fourier analysis. Despite the multitude of factors that contribute to corneal power, the cornea has been characterized by the single K-value from the earliest IOL formulae to those more recently like the Olsen and Holladay.[2] This K-number represents an arbitrary paraxial corneal power using an assumptive corneal index of refraction due to the absence of data concerning the posterior corneal power with routine biometry. This works reasonably well for regular corneas where the assumptions that are made regarding the RI and the posterior corneal curvature are relatively accurate. In these corneas, HOAs do not play a major role and their contribution to the refractive power of the cornea is almost negligible. Ray-tracing modeling has confirmed these findings too: Okulix (Tedics Peric & Jöher) and PhacoOptics (IOL Innovations) use thick-lens models and can further calculate spherical aberration. Newer devices like the Sirius tomographer (CSO) use ray tracing with a thick-lens model to predict ELP and they do not assume total corneal power, but rather measure the posterior cornea directly and then calculate the total corneal power.

17.2 Biometry in Irregular Corneas

These corneas have high degrees of HOAs and the typical anterior cornea: posterior cornea curvature relationship (Gullstrand's ratio) can be distorted. Additionally, the devices measuring these corneas are also affected by the irregularity. Keep in mind that the posterior corneal surface is imaged through the irregular anterior surface that due to its irregularity will affect the quality of the posterior corneal data. Additionally, the RI of the cornea continues to be an assumption and is not directly measured. The most common irregular corneas encountered are those following previous corneal refractive surgery, corneal scars, dry eye, and keratoconus. It is critical to mention dry eye here as it will impact the quality of the biometry corneal data and the topographic data. Correct diagnosis of the corneal condition is paramount as different conditions will affect the calculation process differently. Examining the corneal topography is critical and biometry alone does not suffice. Corneal HOAs are also measured and quantified and are normally around $0.40 \pm 0.15\,\mu m^2$. Higher levels than this indicate some level of corneal irregularity. In keratoconus, the most important HOA is normally vertical coma and most keratoconus corneas are also hyperprolate inducing abnormally high levels of negative spherical aberration. As with all corneal irregularities or whole eye wavefront measurements, pupil size directly impacts the total HOA level—the larger the pupil, the greater the HOAs. Fortunately, following cataract surgery, pupil size is often smaller and typically between 4.0 and 5.0 mm and thus HOAs (by convention measured at 6.0 mm) are less relevant. As previously mentioned, RGP CLs can also be very valuable to assess the corneal contribution to the reduced visual acuity when corrected distance visual acuity (CDVA) appears to be less than expected given the density of the cataract and the retinal health.

In keratoconus specifically, a problem of optical decentration exists, but it is different to the decentration that we deal with following decentered corneal ablative refractive procedures. In keratoconus, the posterior cornea steepens along with the anterior cornea, decreasing the anterior-to-posterior ratio (A-P ratio; unlike in ablative corneal surgery where the posterior corneal curvature typically remains unchanged.) This leads to an overestimation of the actual corneal net power. A second factor is the ELP, which is more posterior than in normal eyes due to the anterior displacement of the cornea. Both factors shift the refractive prediction error toward hyperopia. This is the very reason that in mild to moderate keratoconus, a regular vergence formula can be used, targeting mild myopia.

When multifocality within the optically active visual axis is pronounced as with more advanced keratoconus, ray-tracing software should be used to select the best IOL power. If possible, increase the ELP, as there is no algorithm specific for keratoconic eyes. A simple alternative is to target a slightly myopic refraction.

This chapter is specifically about cataract surgery in keratoconic eyes, but having a basic understanding of the methodology of calculating IOL power in other corneal irregular conditions is helpful. The main change after corneal ablative surgery (PRK and laser in situ keratomileusis [LASIK]) and small incision lenticule extraction (SMILE; stromal lenticule removal) is the change of the anterior corneal radius. The posterior corneal radius remains unchanged for the most part. Spherical aberration can be a problem as well as ELP if anterior corneal data only are used to predict it. Vergence formulas that use the double-K method for ELP calculations and use regression analysis to correct the Gullstrand ratio (A-P corneal curvature ratio) can be used here. These include the double-K Sanders–Retzlaff–Kraff (SRK)/T, the Holladay, Haigis-L, Shammas-PL, and the Barrett True-K formulas. Intraoperative biometry also has value[3] to help refine the IOL power choice and toricity, and this applies to keratoconic corneas too.

The findings after radial keratotomy (RK) are different to the ablative techniques. The anterior radius of the cornea is typically flatter than normal. A double-*K* method is critical, as the anterior cornea in these post-RK eyes cannot be used to predict ELP. The key difference, however, when compared to ablative techniques is that the posterior cornea is also flattened, producing a different A-P ratio to an ablative procedure for the same level of refractive correction. The measured *K*-value will underestimate the true corneal power unlike in keratoconus, where it will overestimate the actual corneal power.

Decentered corneal surgery impairs the optical performance of the cornea irrespective of whether it was LASIK, PRK, SMILE, or RK, mainly due to induced coma that can be vertical, horizontal, or oblique. The greater the corneal irregularity, the more it makes sense to use exact optics rather than paraxial optics. The refraction itself is prone to the same issues with the multiple refractive corrections that can be successfully utilized depending on which part of the cornea the patient looks through. Ray tracing has the potential to add value here with the central corneal data being imported into the ray-tracing software and then retinal image quality being assessed with direct ray tracing assuming different power IOLs in the model.

17.3 Intraocular Lens Considerations

17.3.1 Toric Lenses

IOL power is the main aim of biometry and in patients with corneal astigmatism, toric IOLs have a significant role to play in improving UDVA. With keratoconus, the astigmatism is frequently irregular and selecting a toric IOL is more challenging. This challenge is further complicated when there has been previous corneal surgery like intrastromal corneal rings, corneal collagen crosslinking (CXL) or keratoplasty. Modern toric IOLs have been shown to provide excellent efficacy, predictability, and safety when used to correct corneal astigmatism during cataract and refractive lens exchange surgery in normal eyes, especially in eyes with more than 1.5 diopters of astigmatism. There is a paucity of peer-reviewed articles on toric IOLs in keratoconus, however.[4,5,6,7,8,9,10,11,12,13]

There are also some theoretical concerns about the use of toric lenses with high levels of cylinder. Some companies manufacture lenses to order and can deliver customized lenses with very high cylinders. The optical performance of high-magnitude toric lenses can be influenced based on whether the lens astigmatism is on a single surface, often the back or "bitoric," whereby astigmatism is split and shared on the front and back surfaces (AT Torbi, Zeiss, Jena, Germany).

Another concern is understanding the axis to use for toric lens alignment. Often the axis of astigmatism is nonorthogonal and asymmetric and the true alignment axis is based on the vector analysis considering the magnitude of astigmatism at each meridian. One of the authors (SD) has for over 10 years used the axis of the S2 aberration for astigmatism derived from corneal topography to align toric lenses and has found this to be a very useful and accurate method in keratoconus and form fruste keratoconus (▶ Fig. 17.2). The magnitude of astigmatism at the cornea can also contribute to the decision-making process of the amount of astigmatism that might wish to be considered when planning the procedure. Again in one of the author's (SD) experience, correction beyond 6.0 diopters can lead to problems from abnormal optics as well as increased error in terms of calculation and residual astigmatism if misaligned by even small levels normally considered within tolerance (±5 degrees).

In keratoconus, the visual axis is typically along the slope of the cone and not at the apex of the cornea (except with central keratoconus) and hence *K*-readings may be falsely high for biometry purposes. The software employed in the IOL calculators was validated on normal eyes and will not necessarily transfer to keratoconus eyes either. Most normal eyes show the corneal apex being coincidental with the visual axis.[8] It makes sense therefore to use toric IOLs in eyes with stable mild to moderate keratoconus with relatively regular central corneal astigmatism.

17.4 Other Intraocular Lens Options

An exciting lens option for use in keratoconus is the IC8 Lens (AcuFocus). This is a small-aperture lens designed to provide increased depth of focus and works on the principle of the pinhole. The benefit of the use of this lens is the pinhole effect also reduces the impact of corneal astigmatism as well as irregularity,[14] both of relevance in keratoconus. Kermani implanted the lens unilaterally in four patients and bilaterally in two patients with keratoconus with unaided visual acuities of 6/12

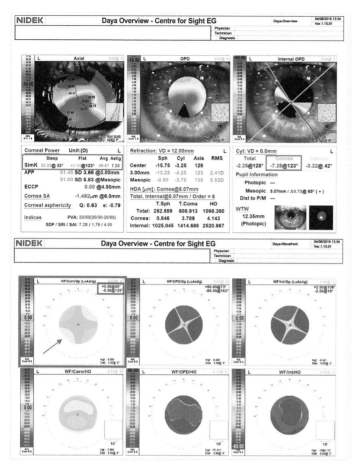

Fig. 17.2 OPD-Scan III (Nidek) report showing the corneal astigmatic aberrations (S2) with an indication of magnitude and axis. The left-hand column shows the corneal topography and simulated K readings outlined with astigmatism of 7.25 diopters at a positive axis of 33 degrees. The image toward the bottom outlined in purple shows corneal astigmatism as derived from corneal topography with a magnitude of 5.50 diopters at a plus axis of 45 degrees and the arrow showing the positive axis.

or better in all cases along with improved unaided near vision (personal communication). Additionally, his colleague Georg Gerten, MD, implanted an IC8 lens in a patient with keratoconus that had previous intracorneal rings placed and obtained a very good visual outcome.[15]

17.4.1 Cataract Surgery: Technical Aspects

Preventing surgically induced astigmatism (SIA) is paramount in keratoconic eyes. The use of MICS (micro-incisional cataract surgery with incisions less than 2.2 mm) may be preferable as incisions larger than this may result in unpredictable outcomes in these eyes.[16,17,18] The smaller the incision and more posterior, the better in these already weakened corneas. Large incisions would induce larger than typically encountered SIA. Some toric calculators use a fixed ratio for cylinder at IOL plane and cylinder at the corneal plane. This is likely to

fail as the ELP is going to impact both the IOL spherical and toric power. Vertex formulae should be used to calculate the IOL power required in the IOL plane.

17.5 Results of Cataract Surgery in Keratoconic Eyes

Good outcomes are achievable especially if a few specific guidelines are followed. Nanavaty et al reported excellent outcomes with 75% of eyes seeing 20/40 or 6/12 (0.5) UDVA and a reduction in cylinder from 3.00 ± 1.00 to 0.70 ± 0.80 diopter cylinder (DC).[8] Outcomes reported by Leccisotti were not quite as good following clear lens extraction/refractive lens exchange (CLE/RLE) and toric IOL implantation. Thirty-two percent or 11 eyes required IOL exchange. At 12 months postoperative, the mean sphere equivalent was −1.31 ± 1.08 diopters and the safety index was 1.38, while the

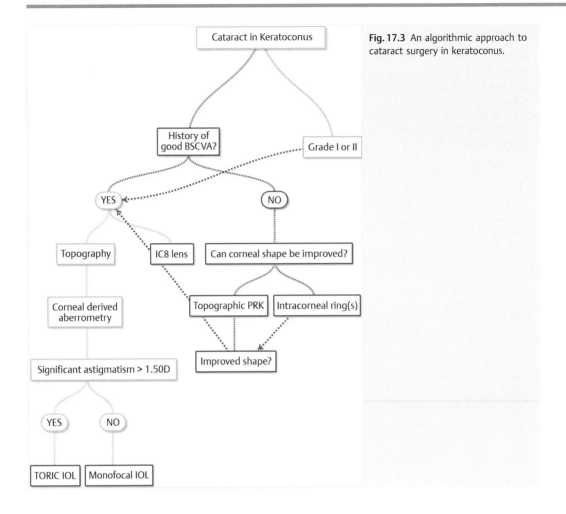

Fig. 17.3 An algorithmic approach to cataract surgery in keratoconus.

efficacy was 0.87.[19] In a case series with 19 eyes SE decreased from –5.25 ± 6.40 diopters preoperatively to +0.22 ± 1.01 diopters postoperatively. Cylinder changed from 3.95 ±1.30 to 1.36 ±1.17 DC postoperatively ($p < 0.01$).[10]

Alió and colleagues published the largest series of MICS with toric IOL implantation in keratoconic eyes.[13] This included 17 eyes. Statistically significant improvements were seen in cylinder reduction, defocus equivalent, and UDVA and CDVA. The MICS approach ensured that keratometry was unchanged. Sixty percent (nine eyes) achieved postoperative UDVA of 20/30 or better. Efficacy was 1.17 ± 0.66 and safety was 1.38 ± 0.58. These results above clearly illustrate that lens removal and toric IOL implantation can demonstrate a statistically significant improvement in UDVA, CDVA, cylinder, efficacy, and safety but that the results are not as good as are typically obtained in cataract or CLE in normal corneas.

17.6 Conclusion

In undertaking cataract surgery in the presence of keratoconus, an algorithmic approach may be useful (▶ Fig. 17.3). Cataract surgery in keratoconic eyes requires considerably more preoperative planning and consideration. The procedure is successful and can lead to very satisfactory outcomes. Improvement in vision and in quality of life typically ensues but the approach is different to cataract or CLE surgery in eyes with normal corneas. Patient selection is key, additional efforts need to be made in terms of IOL calculations using topography to assist biometry, the use of MICS rather than larger incisions, and the selective use of toric and other IOLs.

17.7 Key Pearls

- In advanced keratoconus, ray-tracing software should be used to select the best IOL power and it is always beneficial to target a slightly myopic refraction.
- The use of toric IOLs and a specially designed IC8 Lens (AcuFocus) that is a small-aperture lens designed to provide increased depth of focus and works on the principle of the pinhole is effective in cases of keratoconus.
- The surgical incision should be placed away from the cornea and an MICS would be preferred, as it tends to have a smaller incision with reduced chances of inducing SIA.

References

[1] Belin MW, Duncan JK. Keratoconus: the ABCD grading system. Klin Monatsbl Augenheilkd. 2016; 233(6):701–707

[2] Read SA, Collins MJ, Iskander DR, Davis BA. Corneal topography with Scheimpflug imaging and videokeratography: comparative study of normal eyes. J Cataract Refract Surg. 2009; 35(6):1072–1081

[3] Ianchulev T, Hoffer KJ, Yoo SH, et al. Intraoperative refractive biometry for predicting intraocular lens power calculation after prior myopic refractive surgery. Ophthalmology. 2014; 121(1):56–60

[4] Visser N, Gast ST, Bauer NJ, Nuijts RM. Cataract surgery with toric intraocular lens implantation in keratoconus: a case report. Cornea. 2011; 30(6):720–723

[5] Visser N, Bauer NJ, Nuijts RM. Toric intraocular lenses: historical overview, patient selection, IOL calculation, surgical techniques, clinical outcomes, and complications. J Cataract Refract Surg. 2013; 39(4):624–637

[6] Thebpatiphat N, Hammersmith KM, Rapuano CJ, Ayres BD, Cohen EJ. Cataract surgery in keratoconus. Eye Contact Lens. 2007; 33(5):244–246

[7] Statham M, Apel A, Stephensen D. Comparison of the AcrySof SA60 spherical intraocular lens and the AcrySof Toric SN60T3 intraocular lens outcomes in patients with low amounts of corneal astigmatism. Clin Experiment Ophthalmol. 2009; 37 (8):775–779

[8] Nanavaty MA, Lake DB, Daya SM. Outcomes of pseudophakic toric intraocular lens implantation in Keratoconic eyes with cataract. J Refract Surg. 2012; 28(12):884–889

[9] Lee SJ, Kwon HS, Koh IH. Sequential intrastromal corneal ring implantation and cataract surgery in a severe keratoconus patient with cataract. Korean J Ophthalmol. 2012; 26(3): 226–229

[10] Jaimes M, Xacur-García F, Alvarez-Melloni D, Graue-Hernández EO, Ramirez-Luquín T, Navas A. Refractive lens exchange with toric intraocular lenses in keratoconus. J Refract Surg. 2011; 27(9):658–664

[11] Holland E, Lane S, Horn JD, Ernest P, Arleo R, Miller KM. The AcrySof Toric intraocular lens in subjects with cataracts and corneal astigmatism: a randomized, subject-masked, parallel-group, 1-year study. Ophthalmology. 2010; 117(11): 2104–2111

[12] Ernest P, Potvin R. Effects of preoperative corneal astigmatism orientation on results with a low-cylinder-power toric intraocular lens. J Cataract Refract Surg. 2011; 37(4):727–732

[13] Alió JL, Peña-García P, Abdulla Guliyeva F, Soria FA, Zein G, Abu-Mustafa SK. MICS with toric intraocular lenses in keratoconus: outcomes and predictability analysis of postoperative refraction. Br J Ophthalmol. 2014; 98(3):365–370

[14] Schultz T, Dick HB. Small-aperture intraocular lens implantation in a patient with an irregular cornea. J Refract Surg. 2016; 32(10):706–708

[15] Kermani O.. The challenge of keratoconus in cataract surgery and the benefits of a small-aperture IOL. Cataract Refract Surg Today Europe. 2017

[16] Oshika T, Nagahara K, Yaguchi S, et al. Three year prospective, randomized evaluation of intraocular lens implantation through 3.2 and 5.5 mm incisions. J Cataract Refract Surg. 1998; 24(4):509–514

[17] Masket S, Wang L, Belani S. Induced astigmatism with 2.2- and 3.0-mm coaxial phacoemulsification incisions. J Refract Surg. 2009; 25(1):21–24

[18] Kohnen T, Dick B, Jacobi KW. Comparison of the induced astigmatism after temporal clear corneal tunnel incisions of different sizes. J Cataract Refract Surg. 1995; 21(4):417–424

[19] Leccisotti A. Refractive lens exchange in keratoconus. J Cataract Refract Surg. 2006; 32(5):742–746

18 Bilensectomy (Phakic IOL Explantation with Coincidental Cataract Surgery and IOL Implantation)

Veronica Vargas Fragoso and Jorge L. Alió

Abstract

Phakic intraocular lenses (IOLs) are a useful tool in the armamentarium of a refractive surgeon, especially in those patients in which corneal refractive surgery cannot be performed. Although an excellent visual outcome is achieved after the implantation of phakic IOLs, they need to be explanted at some point of time due to the development of cataract (in most of the cases). There are three types of phakic IOLs: angle supported, iris fixated, and posterior chamber IOLs. Angle-supported IOLs are no longer used due to the complications that they are associated with (severe endothelial cell loss, pupil ovalization). Before performing bilensectomy, a careful examination must be done to manage possible complications during and after surgery; for example, the presence of posterior synechiae, a low endothelial cell count, severe pupil ovalization, or a poor mydriasis. A fundus examination in these patients is also very important because many of them are high myopes with long axial lengths that are susceptible to retinal detachments. The aim of this chapter is to discuss the main uses of bilensectomy and describe the surgical technique (which is going to be different depending on the type of phakic IOL) and the visual outcomes.

Keywords: bilensectomy, phakic intraocular lens, cataract, micro-incisional cataract surgery (MICS), endothelial cell loss, posterior synechiae

18.1 Introduction

The term bilensectomy was first introduced by Joseph Collins and refers to the explantation of a phakic intraocular lens (IOL), followed by phacoemulsification and implantation of a posterior chamber IOL.[1] Placement of phakic IOL can lead to corneal endothelial decompensation along with cataract formation. Although the removal of phakic IOL becomes mandatory in such cases, the potential outcomes can be limited or restricted in nature due to associated clinical features and decompensation. These cases need a particular mention that the decompensated endothelium needs to be protected at all stages of surgical maneuver and in advanced cases it may also be essential to perform an endothelial keratoplasty procedure.

18.1.1 Phakic Intraocular Lenses

There are three types of phakic IOLs:
- Angle supported.
- Iris fixated.
- Posterior chamber IOLs.

Phakic IOLs have many advantages: they preserve accommodation, they can correct high refractive errors, and they achieve a good visual outcome and optical quality,[2,3] but it is essential to mention that all of them eventually need to be explanted because of the natural development of cataract.[4] In fact, cataract is the main cause of phakic IOL explantation in all types of phakic IOLs,[5] with posterior chamber phakic IOLs reporting the highest rate of cataract formation,[5] which may be due to an improper vaulting, chronic inflammation secondary to friction between the IOL and iris, and/or inadequate aqueous perfusion to the lens.[3] Also, the use of steroids, trauma during surgery, and high myopia are important causes of cataract formation independent of the type of phakic IOL implanted.[5]

18.1.2 Indications of Bilensectomy

- When the corrected distance visual acuity (CDVA) has decreased at least two lines from the CDVA measured after phakic IOL implantation and the loss of vision is related to cataract formation.
- When there is a functional loss of endothelial cell count (< 1,500 cells/mm^2).
- Significant pupil ovalization in patients older than 45 years (▶ Fig. 18.1).[1,5]

▶ Table 18.1 lists the main causes of phakic IOL explantation according to a multicentric study.[5]

18.1.3 Preoperative Evaluation

Anterior chamber depth measurement, the position of the IOL in relation to the corneal

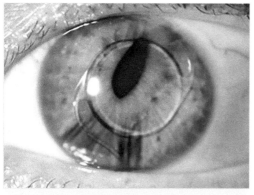

Fig. 18.1 Severe pupil ovalization and iris atrophy in a patient with an angle supported phakic intraocular lens.

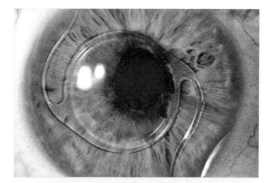

Fig. 18.2 Presence of posterior synechiae in an eye with an angle supported phakic intraocular lens.

Table 18.1 Causes of phakic intraocular lens explantation

Cause of explantation	Angle supported (%)	Iris fixated (%)	Posterior chamber (%)
Cataract	51.39	44.83	65.28
Endothelial cell loss	15.97	8.33	1.39
Corneal decompen-sation	10.42	20.83	2.78
Dislocation	7.64	4.17	5.56
Pupil ovalization	6.25	4.17	0
Retinal detachment	1.39	8.33	4.17
Ocular hypertension	3.47	4.17	8.33
Inadequate size power	2.08	4.17	11.11
Halos and glare	1.39	0	1.39

endothelium, iris, and lens, and the presence of synechiae (▶ Fig. 18.2) has to be evaluated before surgery, as well as the endothelial cell count to prevent corneal decompensation after surgery, and a fundus examination.

18.1.4 Intraocular Lens Calculation

The presence of a phakic IOL does not interfere with the calculation of the pseudophakic IOL.[2] It can be done with ultrasound or optical biometry in phakic mode.

18.2 Surgical Technique

The surgical technique will depend on the type of phakic IOL that has to be explanted, and it can be done with either topical or peribulbar anesthesia depending on the surgeon preferences. During the surgery, the use of high-viscosity viscoelastic to protect the corneal endothelium is mandatory.

18.2.1 Angle-Supported Intraocular Lens

Baikoff (Domilens) IOL: After performing peritomy and cauterization of the vessels, a 6-mm scleral incision is done with a crescent knife 1.5 mm posterior to the limbus. Then, we create a tunnel into the clear cornea, perform two 1-mm side ports, and inject viscoelastic. The IOL is removed carefully and the scleral wound is closed with Nylon 10–0 (▶ Fig. 18.3, ▶ Fig. 18.4) in order to continue with phacoemulsification. A study reported a frequent iris prolapse during surgery using coaxial phacoemulsification, but it was not reported using the micro-incisional cataract surgery (MICS) technique.[1]

Kelman Duet IOL: The first step is to do two 1-mm side ports, followed by the injection of dispersive viscoelastic. The optic is released of the haptic, then a 3-mm clear corneal incision is performed, and the optic is cut with Vannas scissors and explanted with the use of a forceps. The haptic is also explanted through the main incision with a

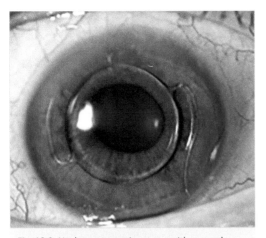

Fig. 18.3 Nuclear cataract in an eye with an angle supported intraocular lens.

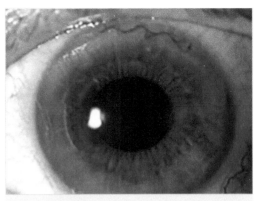

Fig. 18.4 Postoperative image of the eye in ▶ Fig. 18.3 after bilensectomy.

forceps; coaxial or MICS phacoemulsification is performed in a normal fashion.

18.2.2 Iris-Fixated Intraocular Lens

Artisan IOL: The first step is to do a peritomy and a light cauterization of the vessels, a 6-mm curvilinear scleral incision with a crescent knife is done 1.5 mm posterior to the limbus with a depth of 0.3 mm approximately, followed by an anterior dissection parallel to the corneoscleral surface that is done to create a tunnel into the clear cornea. One-millimeter side ports are done, followed by the injection of dispersive viscoelastic to protect the corneal endothelium. With the use of a keratome, enter the anterior chamber through the scleral tunnel and with the Artisan implantation forceps grab the optic of the IOL and with the enclavation needle de-enclavate the haptics. Once the haptics are free, rotate the IOL into a vertical position and pull it out of the anterior chamber. Suture the scleral incision with Nylon 10–0 to proceed with phacoemulsification.

Artiflex IOL: Since the optic of the IOL is made of silicone (polysiloxane), it can be explanted through a 3.2-mm clear corneal incision. The de-enclavation procedure of the haptics is the same as with the Artisan IOL. Before doing the phacoemulsification, liberate the synechiae carefully if any.

18.2.3 Posterior Chamber Phakic Intraocular Lens

ICL: Two 1-mm side ports are created, followed by the injection of intracameral mydriatic and viscoelastic above and underneath the IOL and with the aid of a Sinskey hook, the IOL is moved into the anterior chamber. A 2.8- to 3.2-mm main incision is made and the IOL is rotated in order to have one of the footplates in front of the incision, which is then grabbed and removed with a forceps.[6] The surgeon can then continue with coaxial phacoemulsification or close the main incision and perform MICS phacoemulsification through the two 1-mm side ports.

18.3 Outcomes

In eyes with angle-supported IOLs that had bilensectomy due to pupil ovalization, the surgery has been reported as a more difficult procedure due to the presence of angle adhesions and iris synechia.[1] When bilensectomy was performed secondary to cataract formation, the surgery was without any untoward incidence when it was performed with MICS, whereas when it was performed with coaxial phacoemulsification, iris prolapse was an important issue during surgery. The adhesions between the lens and the iris were not observed in patients who had bilensectomy due to endothelial cell loss.[1] In posterior chamber phakic IOLs, the visual outcomes of bilensectomy are good and predictable,[6] achieving high level of patient satisfaction, and the surgery has been reported as a relatively easy procedure due to the flexibility of the IOL.[7]

18.4 Key Pearls

- Bilensectomy is the term given to the explantation of a phakic IOL, followed by phacoemulsification and implantation of a posterior chamber IOL.
- The presence of a phakic IOL does not interfere in a negative way to the calculation of a pseudophakic IOL power and it can be done with optical biometry.
- The surgical technique will depend on the type of phakic IOL that has to be explanted.
- Good visual and refractive outcomes are achieved after bilensectomy in most cases.

Videos

Video 18.1 Bilensectomy: Kelman's intraocular lens (IOL) explantation. The Duet Kelman phakic IOL is cut and is explanted followed by phacoemulsification procedure to remove the cataractous lens.

Video 18.2 Bilensectomy: Artisan's intraocular lens (IOL) explantation. A scleral tunnel incision is framed and the phakic Artisan IOL is explanted. Synechiolysis is done followed by

phacoemulsification of the dense cataract and a three-piece IOL implantation.

Video 18.3 Implantable contact lens (IPCL) explantation. The IPCL explantation is done from the scleral tunnel wound followed by phacoemulsification and intraocular lens implantation.

References

[1] Alió JL, Abdelrahman AM, Javaloy J, Iradier MT, Ortuño V. Angle-supported anterior chamber phakic intraocular lens explantation causes and outcome. Ophthalmology. 2006; 113 (12):2213–2220

[2] Chen LJ, Chang YJ, Kuo JC, Rajagopal R, Azar DT. Metaanalysis of cataract development after phakic intraocular lens surgery. J Cataract Refract Surg. 2008; 34(7):1181–1200

[3] Moshirfar M, Mifflin M, Wong G, Chang JC. Cataract surgery following phakic intraocular lens implantation. Curr Opin Ophthalmol. 2010; 21(1):39–44

[4] Colin J. Bilensectomy: the implications of removing phakic intraocular lenses at the time of cataract extraction. J Cataract Refract Surg. 2000; 26(1):2–3

[5] Alió JL, Toffaha BT, Peña-Garcia P, Sádaba LM, Barraquer RI. Phakic intraocular lens explantation: causes in 240 cases. J Refract Surg. 2015; 31(1):30–35

[6] Meier PG, Majo F, Othenin-Girard P, Bergin C, Guber I. Refractive outcomes and complications after combined copolymer phakic intraocular lens explantation and phacoemulsification with intraocular lens implantation. J Cataract Refract Surg. 2017; 43(6):748–753

[7] Kamiya K, Shimizu K, Igarashi A, Aizawa D, Ikeda T. Clinical outcomes and patient satisfaction after visian implantable collamer lens removal and phacoemulsification with intraocular lens implantation in eyes with induced cataract. Eye (Lond). 2010; 24(2):304–309

19 Cystoid Macular Edema and Management

J. Fernando Arevalo, Carlos F. Fernández, and Fernando A. Arevalo

Abstract

Cystoid macular edema (CME) is more commonly seen after complicated cataract surgery associated with vitreous loss, but it is also reported following uncomplicated cataract surgery. This chapter deals with the prevention and treatment options that help curtail CME and optimize the postoperative outcomes.

Keywords: cystoid macular edema, Irvine–Gass syndrome, pseudophakic cystoid macular edema, fluorescein angiography, OCT angiography, macular edema

19.1 Introduction

Cystoid macular edema (CME) following cataract surgery was initially reported by Irvine in 1953 and is known as the Irvine–Gass syndrome.[1,2] CME is one of the most common causes of unexpected decreased visual acuity after ophthalmic surgery. Despite recent advances in cataract surgery technique and instrumentation, pseudophakic cystoid macular edema (PCME) occurs most frequently after cataract surgery even after uncomplicated surgery (▸ Fig. 19.1).[3] The incidence of PCME in different cataract extraction techniques in uncomplicated cataract operations are as follows: after intracapsular cataract extraction 8%, after extracapsular cataract extraction 0.8 to 20%, after phacoemulsification 0.1 to 2.35%, and after femtosecond-assisted cataract surgery 1.18%.[3] CME exhibits dilation of normal retinal capillaries around the fovea, with consequent fluid leakage and microcystoid formation.

19.2 Histology

CME consists of a localized expansion of the retinal intracellular and/or extracellular space in the macular area. This predilection to the macular region is probably associated with the loose binding of inner connecting fibers in Henle's layer, allowing accumulation of fluid leaking from perifoveal capillaries (▸ Fig. 19.2).[4] Recently, Antcliff et al[5] concluded that the inner and outer plexiform layers constitute high-resistance barriers to fluid flow through the retina, which accounts for the characteristic distribution of CME. In CME associated with cataract extraction, the cysts were most prominent in the inner nuclear layer and less prominent in the outer plexiform layer.

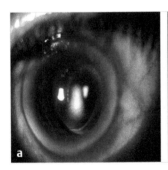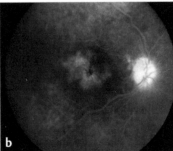

Fig. 19.1 (a) Photography of the anterior segment after uneventful cataract surgery showing a multifocal intraocular lens in the posterior chamber. **(b)** Fluorescein angiography shows pseudophakic cystoid macular edema.

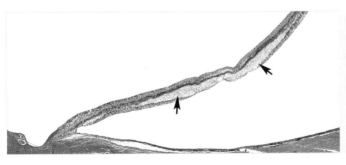

Fig. 19.2 Histology of pseudophakic cystoid macular edema showing cystic spaces in the outer plexiform layer (*black arrows*). Retinal detachment is an artifact. (These images are provided courtesy of Dr. Deepak Edward.)

19.3 Pathogenesis

Several theories exist regarding the pathogenesis of CME.[6,7] The theories involve changes in the perifoveal retina where the vascular permeability of the retinal capillaries is altered, leading to leakage of plasma into the central retina, which causes it to thicken because of excess interstitial fluid. The excess interstitial fluid is likely to disrupt ion fluxes, and the thickening of the macula results in stretching and distortion of neurons. There is reversible reduction in visual acuity, but over time the perturbed neurons die, which results in permanent visual loss (▶ Fig. 19.3).[8,9,10,11,12,13]

Cataract surgery in diabetic patients may result in a dramatic acceleration of preexisting diabetic macular edema leading to poor functional visual outcome (▶ Fig. 19.4). This can be prevented provided the severity of the retinopathy is recognized preoperatively and treated appropriately with prompt laser photocoagulation either before surgery, if there is adequate fundal view, or shortly afterward.

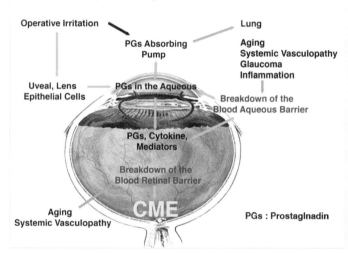

Hypothesis on Pathogenesis of Pseudophakic Cystoid Macular Edema

Operative Irritation

PGs Absorbing Pump

Uveal, Lens Epithelial Cells

PGs in the Aqueous

PGs, Cytokine, Mediators

Breakdown of the Blood Retinal Barrier

CME

Aging Systemic Vasculopathy

Lung

Aging Systemic Vasculopathy Glaucoma Inflammation

Breakdown of the Blood Aqueous Barrier

PGs : Prostaglnadin

Fig. 19.3 Inflammatory hypothesis on the pathogenesis of pseudophakic cystoid macular edema. (Adapted from Miyake K, Ibaraki N. Prostaglandins and cystoid macular edema. Surv Ophthalmol 2002;47 (suppl 1):S203–S218)

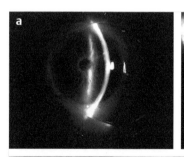
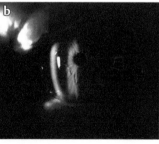
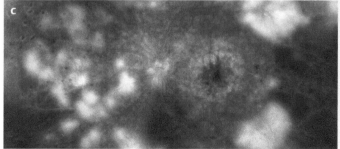

Fig. 19.4 (a) Photograph of the anterior segment after uneventful phacoemulsification cataract surgery showing anterior chamber fibrin in a patient with diabetes. (b) Photograph of the anterior segment post-treatment with tissue plasminogen activator in the anterior chamber showing disappearance of the fibrin. (c) Fluorescein angiography after cataract surgery showing macular edema and proliferative diabetic retinopathy.

19.3.1 Natural History

Approximately 20% of the patients who undergo uncomplicated phacoemulsification or extracapsular extraction develop angiographically proven CME. However, a clinically significant decrease in visual acuity is seen only in about 1% of these eyes. Spontaneous resolution of the CME with subsequent visual improvement may occur within 3 to 12 months in 80% of the patients. Chronic CME is defined as a persistent decline in visual acuity for more than 6 months. Interestingly, complicated cataract extraction is associated with an increased risk for clinically significant CME, such as disruption of the anterior vitreous hyaloid (▶ Fig. 19.5), vitreous loss, retention of lens cortex, vitreous strands to the wound (▶ Fig. 19.6), dislocated intraocular lens (IOL), inadequate wound closure, and chronic inflammation[14] and in patients with significant postoperative inflammation.

19.4 Clinical Presentation

PCME should be suspected when a patient without underlying risk factors complains of decreased vision or metamorphopsia following cataract extraction. Clinically, intraretinal edema contained in cystlike spaces in a honeycomb pattern around the fovea can be seen. Diagnosis is based on the clinical findings and characteristic appearance on fundus fluorescein angiography and optical coherence tomography (OCT).

The fluorescein angiography pattern is characteristic. Early phases of fluorescein angiography demonstrate dye leakage from the parafoveal retinal capillaries, and later phases of the angiogram demonstrate the petaloid pattern of leakage into the parafoveal intraretinal spaces along with optic disc hyperfluorescence (▶ Fig. 19.7).

OCT is a sensitive noninvasive tool that can clearly demonstrate these cystoid spaces as well as

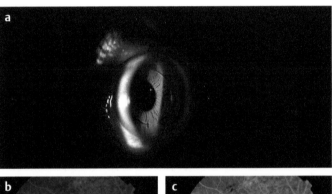
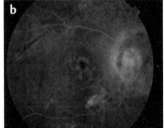
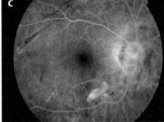

Fig. 19.5 (a) Photograph of the anterior segment showing anterior chamber intraocular lens because of vitreous loss and posterior capsule rupture. (b) Fluorescein angiography showing pseudophakic cystoid macular edema. (c) Fluorescein angiography showing the resolution of the cystoid macular edema after intravitreal bevacizumab.

Fig. 19.6 (a) Photograph of the anterior segment showing vitreous strands to the wound. (b) Fluorescein angiography showing cystoid macular edema.

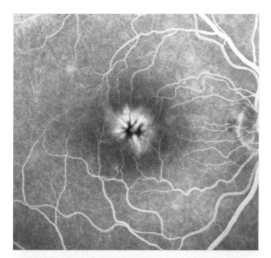

Fig. 19.7 Fluorescein angiography showing the classic petaloid appearance in a patient with pseudophakic cystoid macular edema.

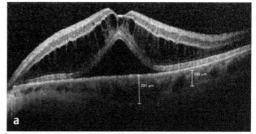

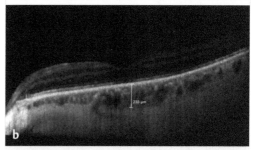

Fig. 19.8 **(a)** Spectral-domain optical coherence tomography can be used to describe the ultrastructural changes; it can show an increased thickness of the fovea and presence of large cystoid spaces in the outer plexiform layer with stretching of the Müller cell processes. In addition, it can show neurosensory retinal detachment and increase in choroidal thickness. **(b)** Re-saturation of the macular anatomy after Aflibercept treatment.

calculate central macular thickness and total macular volume. Spectral-domain OCT (SD-OCT) can show an increased thickness of the fovea and presence of large cystoid spaces in the outer plexiform layer with stretching of the Müller cell processes. OCT can also show increased thickness of the outer nuclear layer. Photoreceptor layer (as represented by inner segment–outer segment line [IS-OS line]) can be intact and the continuity of the external limiting membrane (ELM) can be maintained (▶ Fig. 19.8). Choroidal thickness is increased and decreases following edema resolution. These findings may strengthen the hypothesis of an inflammatory pathogenesis in PCME. Optical coherence tomography angiography (OCT-A) shows capillary changes in PCME; the deep capillary plexus is mainly altered and disorganized with a significant decrease of capillary density in the acute phase of PCME. After macular edema resolution, the pattern of deep capillary plexus recovers and the capillary density returns to normal.

19.5 Prevention

The prophylactic use of nonsteroidal anti-inflammatory drugs (NSAIDs) reduces the incidence of PCME.[15,16,17,18,19,20] The efficacy of prophylactic nonsteroidal anti-inflammatory therapy is greatest when started at 1 or 3 days before surgery, and continued postoperatively for several weeks. Topical NSAIDs are more effective than topical corticosteroids in preventing CME.[21,22]

19.6 Treatment Options

The primary goal of postsurgical CME treatment is to improve visual acuity by decreasing the amount of macular edema once it has formed.

19.6.1 Nonsteroidal Anti-inflammatory Agents

NSAIDs are cyclooxygenase inhibitors that work by preventing the synthesis of prostaglandins. Topical ketorolac tromethamine (Acular) demonstrates a sustained beneficial effect on the visual acuity of treated patients with PCME. Newer-generation NSAIDs, such as bromfenac sodium (Xibrom) and nepafenac, have modifications to their chemical structure, increasing their ocular penetration and theoretical potency.[22,23]

19.6.2 Corticosteroids

Corticosteroid drugs inhibit the leukotrienes and prostaglandins synthesis pathway. In addition to

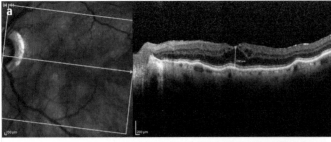

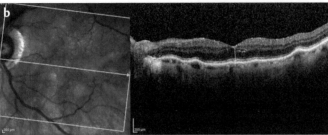

Fig. 19.9 (a) Spectral-domain optical coherence tomography (OCT) showing cystoid macular edema. **(b)** OCT after treatment with intravitreal triamcinolone acetonide with resolution of the cystoid macular edema.

their anti-inflammatory properties, corticosteroids also inhibit macrophage and neutrophil migration and decrease capillary permeability and vasodilation. Corticosteroids are the most common anti-inflammatory treatment after cataract surgery around the world.[24]

19.6.3 Corticosteroid Injections

Some studies have demonstrated the usefulness of an intravitreal (IVT) injection of triamcinolone acetate in the reduction of PCME (▶ Fig. 19.9).[25,26] In order to mitigate the cumulative risk associated with repeated IVT injections, extended-release steroid implants have been investigated for the treatment of macular edema. The three sustained-release corticosteroid implants currently available include Ozurdex (Allergan Inc., Irvine, CA), which releases dexamethasone, and Retisert (Bausch and Lomb, Rochester, NY) and Iluvien (Alimera Science, Alpharetta, GA), both of which release fluocinolone acetonide. However, long-acting steroid preparations have potential side effects such as glaucoma, which is more likely to occur when treatment exceeds 6 months.[27]

19.6.4 Antivascular Endothelial Growth Factor Agents

Surgical trauma leads to post-op inflammation, which can lead to PCME through an increase in the production of vasopermeable factors such as

vascular endothelial growth factor (VEGF). VEGF has been associated with breakdown of the blood–retinal barrier, and contributes to the onset of macular edema. Recent studies showed elevated levels of VEGF and interleukin-6 in ocular fluids of patients with macular edema.[28]

Bevacizumab (Avastin; Genentech, Inc., San Francisco, CA) is a complete full-length humanized antibody that binds to all subtypes of VEGF-A. Recent studies have demonstrated the usefulness of an IVT injection of bevacizumab in the reduction of refractory PCME.[28,29,30,31,32] Other anti-VEGF agents that could be used are ranibizumab and aflibercept.[32]

19.6.5 Vitrectomy

Pars plana vitrectomy with membrane peeling may be considered in cases of PCME with a mechanical component as identified either on clinical examination or by OCT, or in cases of chronic refractory edema unresponsive to medical therapy.[33,34]

19.6.6 Neodymium:Yttrium Aluminum Garnet Vitreolysis

PCME with vitreous incarceration in the corneoscleral wound responds more slowly than without vitreous incarceration. There are several reports of the neodymium:yttrium aluminum garnet (Nd:YAG) vitreolysis being effective in the resolution of PCME in selected patients with vitreous incarceration.[35]

19.6.7 Future Directions

As mentioned earlier, corticosteroids work at the beginning of the inflammatory cascade. Triesence (Alcon Labs, Fort Worth, TX), triamcinolone acetonide for IVT injection during surgery, may be used off-label in the treatment algorithm of recalcitrant PCME. Wu et al[36] reported short-term structural and functional outcomes following IVT injection of infliximab in eyes with refractory PCME treated previously with topical nepafenac 0.1%, topical prednisolone acetate 1%, IVT triamcinolone (4 mg), and IVT bevacizumab (1.25 mg). Most patients experienced best-corrected visual acuity (BCVA) improvement by at least ≥ 3 lines at the 6-month follow-up. BCVA deterioration was not reported in any case.

19.7 Conclusion

Current management includes nonsteroidal anti-inflammatory agents, NSAIDs plus corticosteroids, corticosteroid injections, carbonic anhydrase inhibition, anti-VEGF agents, vitrectomy, and Nd:YAG vitreolysis. New technology has and will revolutionize the diagnosis, prognosis, and treatment of this condition.

19.8 Key Pearls

- Of the various causes and risk factors, vitreomacular traction is a common factor that results into CME due to breakage of blood–retinal barrier leading to leakage and edema.
- OCT examination is often diagnostic in cases with CME with the measurement of retinal thickening and depiction of intraretinal cysts.
- Medical therapy comprises NSAIDs, corticosteroids, anti-VEGF agents, and pharmacological vitreolysis agents.
- Surgical treatment mainly comprises pars plana vitrectomy and peeling of the internal limiting membrane.

References

[1] Irvine SR. A newly defined vitreous syndrome following cataract surgery. Am J Ophthalmol. 1953; 36(5):599–619

[2] Gass JD, Norton EW. Follow-up study of cystoid macular edema following cataract extraction. Trans Am Acad Ophthalmol Otolaryngol. 1969; 73(4):665–682

[3] Grzybowski A, Sikorski BL, Ascaso FJ, Huerva V. Pseudophakic cystoid macular edema: update 2016. Clin Interv Aging. 2016; 11:1221–1229

[4] Tso MO. Pathology of cystoid macular edema. Ophthalmology. 1982; 89(8):902–915

[5] Antcliff RJ, Hussain AA, Marshall J. Hydraulic conductivity of fixed retinal tissue after sequential excimer laser ablation: barriers limiting fluid distribution and implications for cystoid macular edema. Arch Ophthalmol. 2001; 119(4):539–544

[6] Flach AJ. The incidence, pathogenesis and treatment of cystoid macular edema following cataract surgery. Trans Am Ophthalmol Soc. 1998; 96:557–634

[7] Stark WJ, Jr, Maumenee AE, Fagadau W, et al. Cystoid macular edema in pseudophakia. Surv Ophthalmol. 1984; 28 suppl:442–451

[8] Nguyen QD, Tatlipinar S, Shah SM, et al. Vascular endothelial growth factor is a critical stimulus for diabetic macular edema. Am J Ophthalmol. 2006; 142(6):961–969

[9] Foos RY. Posterior vitreous detachment. Trans Am Acad Ophthalmol Otolaryngol. 1972; 76(2):480–497

[10] Miyake K, Ibaraki N. Prostaglandins and cystoid macular edema. Surv Ophthalmol. 2002; 47 suppl 1:S203–S218

[11] Yannuzzi LA. A perspective on the treatment of aphakic cystoid macular edema. Surv Ophthalmol. 1984; 28 suppl:540–553

[12] Jampol LM, Sanders DR, Kraff MC. Prophylaxis and therapy of aphakic cystoid macular edema. Surv Ophthalmol. 1984; 28 suppl:535–539

[13] Foster RE, Lowder CY, Meisler DM, Zakov ZN. Extracapsular cataract extraction and posterior chamber intraocular lens implantation in uveitis patients. Ophthalmology. 1992; 99(8):1234–1241

[14] Spaide RF, Yannuzzi LA, Sisco LJ. Chronic cystoid macular edema and predictors of visual acuity. Ophthalmic Surg. 1993; 24(4):262–267

[15] Henderson BA, Kim JY, Ament CS, Ferrufino-Ponce ZK, Grabowska A, Cremers SL. Clinical pseudophakic cystoid macular edema. Risk factors for development and duration after treatment. J Cataract Refract Surg. 2007; 33(9):1550–1558

[16] Yavas GF, Oztürk F, Küsbeci T. Preoperative topical indomethacin to prevent pseudophakic cystoid macular edema. J Cataract Refract Surg. 2007; 33(5):804–807

[17] McColgin AZ, Raizman MB. Efficacy of topical Voltaren in reducing the incidence of postoperative cystoid macular edema. Invest Ophthalmol Vis Sci. 1999; 40:S289

[18] Wittpenn JR, Silverstein S, Heier J, Kenyon KR, Hunkeler JD, Earl M, Acular LS for Cystoid Macular Edema (ACME) Study Group. A randomized, masked comparison of topical ketorolac 0.4% plus steroid vs steroid alone in low-risk cataract surgery patients. Am J Ophthalmol. 2008; 146(4):554–560

[19] Wolf EJ, Braunstein A, Shih C, Braunstein RE. Incidence of visually significant pseudophakic macular edema after uneventful phacoemulsification in patients treated with nepafenac. J Cataract Refract Surg. 2007; 33(9):1546–1549

[20] Flach AJ, Stegman RC, Graham J, Kruger LP. Prophylaxis of aphakic cystoid macular edema without corticosteroids. A paired-comparison, placebo-controlled double-masked study. Ophthalmology. 1990; 97(10):1253–1258

[21] Kim SJ, Patel SN, Sternberg P, Jr. Routine use of nonsteroidal anti-inflammatory drugs with corticosteroids in cataract surgery: beneficial or redundant? Ophthalmology. 2016; 123(3):444–446

[22] Kessel L, Tendal B, Jørgensen KJ, et al. Post-cataract prevention of inflammation and macular edema by steroid and

nonsteroidal anti-inflammatory eye drops: a systematic review. Ophthalmology. 2014; 121(10):1915–1924

[23] Walters T, Raizman M, Ernest P, Gayton J, Lehmann R. In vivo pharmacokinetics and in vitro pharmacodynamics of nepafenac, amfenac, ketorolac, and bromfenac. J Cataract Refract Surg. 2007; 33(9):1539–1545

[24] Heier JS, Topping TM, Baumann W, Dirks MS, Chern S. Ketorolac versus prednisolone versus combination therapy in the treatment of acute pseudophakic cystoid macular edema. Ophthalmology. 2000; 107(11):2034–2038, discussion 2039

[25] Koutsandrea C, Moschos MM, Brouzas D, Loukianou E, Apostolopoulos M, Moschos M. Intraocular triamcinolone acetonide for pseudophakic cystoid macular edema: optical coherence tomography and multifocal electroretinography study. Retina. 2007; 27(2):159–164

[26] Boscia F, Furino C, Dammacco R, Ferreri P, Sborgia L, Sborgia C. Intravitreal triamcinolone acetonide in refractory pseudophakic cystoid macular edema: functional and anatomic results. Eur J Ophthalmol. 2005; 15(1):89–95

[27] Liu Q, He M, Shi H, et al. Efficacy and safety of different doses of a slow-release corticosteroid implant for macular edema: meta-analysis of randomized controlled trials. Drug Des Devel Ther. 2015; 9:2527–2535

[28] Noma H, Minamoto A, Funatsu H, et al. Intravitreal levels of vascular endothelial growth factor and interleukin-6 are correlated with macular edema in branch retinal vein occlusion. Graefes Arch Clin Exp Ophthalmol. 2006; 244(3):309–315

[29] Arevalo JF, Garcia-Amaris RA, Roca JA, et al. Pan-American Collaborative Retina Study Group. Primary intravitreal bevacizumab for the management of pseudophakic cystoid macular edema: pilot study of the Pan-American Collaborative Retina Study Group. J Cataract Refract Surg. 2007; 33(12):2098–2105

[30] Barone A, Russo V, Prascina F, Delle Noci N. Short-term safety and efficacy of intravitreal bevacizumab for pseudophakic cystoid macular edema. Retina. 2009; 29(1):33–37

[31] Arevalo JF, Maia M, Garcia-Amaris RA, et al. Pan-American Collaborative Retina Study Group. Intravitreal bevacizumab for refractory pseudophakic cystoid macular edema: the Pan-American Collaborative Retina Study Group results. Ophthalmology. 2009; 116(8):1481–1487, 1487.e1

[32] Lin CJ, Tsai YY. Use of Aflibercept for the management of refractory pseudophakic macular edema in Irvine Gass Syndrome and literature review. Retin Cases Brief Rep. 2018; 12(1):59–62

[33] Pendergast SD, Margherio RR, Williams GA, Cox MS, Jr. Vitrectomy for chronic pseudophakic cystoid macular edema. Am J Ophthalmol. 1999; 128(3):317–323

[34] Peyman GA, Canakis C, Livir-Rallatos C, Conway MD. The effect of internal limiting membrane peeling on chronic recalcitrant pseudophakic cystoid macular edema: a report of two cases. Am J Ophthalmol. 2002; 133(4):571–572

[35] Steinert RF, Wasson PJ. Neodymium:YAG laser anterior vitreolysis for Irvine-Gass cystoid macular edema. J Cataract Refract Surg. 1989; 15(3):304–307

[36] Wu L, Arevalo JF, Hernandez-Bogantes E, Roca JA. Intravitreal infliximab for refractory pseudophakic cystoid macular edema: results of the Pan-American Collaborative Retina Study Group. Int Ophthalmol. 2012; 32(3):235–243

20 Endophthalmitis, Toxic Anterior Segment Syndrome, and Vitritis

Andrzej Grzybowski and Magdalena Turczynowska

Abstract

Postoperative endophthalmitis (POE) is one of the most dreadful complications of intraocular surgery. It is crucial to take right and quick decisions in order to achieve optimal clinical results and restore the best possible visual acuity. The differential diagnosis of POE should always be considered; however, in case of any doubt, the patient should be regarded as having infectious endophthalmitis and treated with no delay. The role of preoperative instillation of topical antibiotics as a prophylactic measure for prevention of POE is controversial as it does not have any specific benefit over the usage of chlorhexidine or povidone-iodine preoperatively and intraoperative injection of intracameral antibiotics. The main treatment of POE is injection of intravitreal antibiotics preceded by either vitreous tap biopsy or vitrectomy. The antibiotics of first line of preference are vancomycin (1 mg) and ceftazidime (2 mg). Second choice is a combination of vancomycin (2 mg) and amikacin (400 µg). At the same time, dexamethasone (400 µg) is often administered by intravitreal injection. Toxic anterior chamber syndrome (TASS) can also produce marked sterile inflammation due to toxic substances that enter the anterior chamber during or after surgery. The outbreak of TASS requires thorough analysis of each surgical step and all possible risk factors (especially newly introduced medical substances and devices, its sterilization, storage, and transport conditions) to identify and eradicate the causative agent. There are also various conditions presenting with vitritis, which may mimic as infectious endophthalmitis. They should always be differentiated from endophthalmitis; however, it is important to remember that concomitant endophthalmitis also may be present.

Keywords: intraocular infections, endophthalmitis, toxic anterior segment syndrome, vitritis, postoperative endophthalmitis prophylaxis, antisepsis, antibiotics, intracameral antibiotics, cefuroxime, intravitreal antibiotics, pars plana vitrectomy, endophthalmitis vitrectomy study

20.1 Introduction

Intraocular infections and inflammations are significant complications of cataract surgery, limiting the visual potential of the eye. In severe cases, they can even lead to blindness. Over the recent years, improvements of surgical technology, techniques, and procedures have significantly reduced the incidence of postoperative infections; however, it is impossible to eliminate this problem completely. Therefore, accurate diagnosis and prompt treatment are crucial to achieve optimal clinical results with recovery of useful vision.

20.2 Endophthalmitis

20.2.1 Classification

Endophthalmitis (► Fig. 20.1) is a serious inflammation due to an infectious process from bacteria, fungi, or parasites that enter the eye during the perioperative period. It affects the vitreous cavity and is one of the most dreaded complications of ophthalmic surgery, as it may cause severe visual acuity loss, or even loss of the eye. Endophthalmitis may be divided into several categories depending upon the cause of infection, the onset of symptoms, or the degree of inflammation. Most cases of endophthalmitis are exogenous, and occur after eye surgery (postoperative endophthalmitis [POE]), after penetrating ocular trauma (posttraumatic endophthalmitis), or as an extension of keratitis. Usually POE develops after cataract surgery; however, it can be also a complication of glaucoma surgery (associated with either conjunctival filtering bleb, or glaucoma drainage devices) or intravitreal injections. Endogenous endophthalmitis is an uncommon condition that can arise from bacteremic or fungemic seeding of the eye via the bloodstream. However, endophthalmitis is never a source of bacteremia or fungemia. Common risk factors are intravenous drug abuse, diabetes mellitus, immune compromise, malignancy, and chronic diseases with long hospital stays, catheters, and prolonged intravenous antibiotic

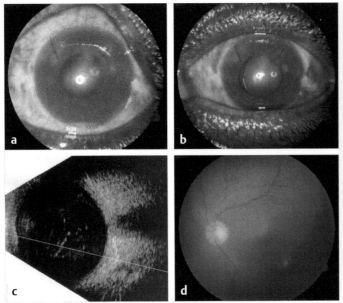

Fig. 20.1 Postoperative endophthalmitis. **(a)** Post cataract extraction, endophthalmitis with corneal clouding, and hypopyon in anterior chamber is noted. **(b)** Post pars plana vitrectomy, cornea clears up with resolving of hypopyon. **(c)** B-scan image depicting the posterior segment involvement with opacities in the vitreous. **(d)** Posterior segment clears up with improved view of the retina and other structures. The vision of the case improved from counting fingers to 20/40 after 2 weeks of performing pars plana vitrectomy.

therapy. The most common pathogens in endophthalmitis vary by category. Most frequently reported organisms causing acute-onset postcataract endophthalmitis are coagulase-negative staphylococci (CNS), whereas *Propionibacterium acnes* usually cause chronic postcataract endophthalmitis. CNS and viridans streptococci are the most common pathogens in endophthalmitis following intravitreal injections, whereas *Streptococcus* species, *Haemophilus influenzae* and *Staphylococcus* species usually cause endophthalmitis following glaucoma surgery. Posttraumatic endophthalmitis, in most of the cases, is caused by *Bacillus* and *Staphylococcus* species. *Candida* species, *Staphylococcus aureus*, and gram-negative bacteria are, in turn, the most common causes of endogenous endophthalmitis. Regardless of category, the most important component of treatment is intravitreal injection of antibiotics, along with vitrectomy in some cases.

20.2.2 Epidemiology

The incidence of postcataract endophthalmitis varies in several countries from 0.03 to 0.7%[1,2,3,4,5,6,7,8,9,10,11,12,13] as presented in ▶ Table 20.1. The recommendations of the European Registry of Quality Outcomes for Cataract and Refractive Surgery (EUREQUO) have set the maximum acceptable level of incidence for POE after cataract extractions as 0.05%.[14] Surgical complications (wound leak, posterior capsule rupture, vitreous loss, or zonular

complications) are related with higher incidence of POE. The elderly patients (older than 85 years), those with clear corneal incisions versus scleral tunnel incisions, and those without intracameral injection of cefuroxime have a higher risk of infection. Moreover, the type of intraocular lens (IOL) implanted is also considered a risk factor. Patients with silicone IOLs have higher probability of endophthalmitis compared to those with acrylic (or other material) IOLs.

20.2.3 Diagnosis

The symptoms of POE vary according to its severity, the most common being pain and visual loss. Patients often demonstrate blurred vision, red eye, swollen eyelids, chemosis, conjunctival injection and discharge, as well as corneal haze, media haze, fibrinous exudate or hypopyon, and vitritis with an impaired view of the fundus. Early recognition leads to better clinical outcomes. The differential diagnosis includes toxic anterior segment syndrome (TASS), retained lens material in the anterior chamber or vitreous, vitreous hemorrhage, postoperative uveitis, and viral retinitis. If there is any doubt about the diagnosis, patients should always be regarded as having infectious endophthalmitis and immediately treated.

Endophthalmitis is initially a clinical diagnosis, and have to be proven by gram stain, culture, or polymerase chain reaction (PCR), although a

Table 20.1 Endophthalmitis rate after cataract surgery in several European countries

Reference	Country	Publication year	Period	Total, N	IPOE, N	IPOE rate (%)	IPOE rate with IC antibiotics	IPOE rate without IC antibiotics (%)
Romero et al[1]	Spain	2006	2001–2004	7,268	25	0.344	0.055% (cefazolin)	0.63
ESCRS[2]	Multiple (9 EU countries)	2007	2003–2005	15,971	20	0.12	0.05% (cefuroxime)	0.35
Yu-Wai-Man et al[3]	United Kingdom	2008	2000–2006	36,743	35	0.095	0.046% (cefuroxime)	0.139
Garat et al[4]	Spain	2009	2002–2007	18,579	31	0.167	0.047% (cefazolin)	0.422
García-Sáenz et al[5]	Spain	2010	1999–2008	13,652	42	0.30	0.590% (cefuroxime)	0.043
Barreau et al[6]	France	2012	2003–2008	5,115	36	0.704	0.044% (cefuroxime)	1.238
Friling et al[7]	Sweden	2013	2005–2010	464,996	135	0.029	0.027% (various)	0.39
Rodríguez-Caravaca et al[8]	Spain	2013	1998–2012	19,463	44	0.23	0.039% (cefuroxime)	0.59
Beselga et al[9]	Portugal	2014	2005–2011	15,689	6	0.038	0.00% (cefuroxime)	0.26
Rahman and Murphy[10]	Ireland	2015	2007–2011	8,239	5	0.061	0.061% (cefuroxime)	–
Lundström et al[11]	Sweden	2015	2001–2010	692,786	244	0.035	0.03% (various, 99% cefuroxime)	0.43
Creuzot-Garcher et al[12]	France	2016	2005–2014	6,371,242	6,668	0.105	0.046–0.111% (cefuroxime)	0.080–0.46%
Daien et al[13]	France	2016	2010–2014	2,434,008	1,941	0.08	0.06% (cefuroxime)	0.09

Abbreviations: IC, intracameral; IPOE, infectious postoperative endophthalmitis.

143

negative culture may occur in up to 30% of cases. This situation does not necessarily rule out the infection and the treatment should be continued. The samples for culture should be obtained from aqueous and vitreous. If the eye media is opaque, the B-scan ultrasound biomicroscopy should be performed to confirm the changes in vitreous and to rule out retinal detachment or other complications that may coexist. An anterior chamber tap should be performed to obtain aqueous sample where 0.1 to 0.2 mL of aqueous is aspirated via limbal paracentesis using a 25-gauge needle. Vitreous samples might be obtained by either needle tap, vitreous biopsy, or pars plana vitrectomy (PPV). The European Society of Cataract and Refractive Surgeons (ESCRS) guidelines favor vitrectomy technique as it allows obtaining larger sample of vitreous, and at the same time removes bacterial load in the vitreous and reduces the need for reoperation.[15] The specimens obtained should be immediately sent to the microbiology laboratory for detailed analysis.

20.2.4 Etiology

Common sources of infection in POE are microorganisms derived from conjunctival sac, contaminated devices, irrigating solutions, the implanted IOL, or airborne contamination. According to the Endophthalmitis Vitrectomy Study (EVS),[16] if only analysis was possible, the intraocular isolates in most cases of patients with bacterial POE were indistinguishable from conjunctival and lid specimens. Microbial spectrum of POE is dependent on environmental, geographical, or climatic factors and varies significantly in different countries.[7,11,17,18,19,20,21,22,23] ▶ Table 20.2 presents the etiology of POE in different regions of the world. In Europe, most commonly isolated organisms in postcataract endophthalmitis are gram-positive bacteria, including *Staphylococcus epidermidis*, *Staphylococcus aureus*, and *Streptococcus pneumoniae*, while gram-negative bacteria are in the minority. However, there are significant differences in a rate of enterococcal infections in Sweden (30–31%) compared with other European countries (2% in the Netherlands and United Kingdom), or the United States (3%).[7,11,17,18,19] This may be connected with extensive use of intracameral cefuroxime in Sweden and increased proportion of cefuroxime-resistant species. In the United States, as in Europe the rate of streptococcal infections is lower, whereas CNS is the most commonly identified microorganism. In tropical regions of Asia, the reported percentage of gram-negative and fungal cases is much higher than in Europe and the United States.[20,21,22,23] It should be emphasized that the main prognostic factor predictive of the final visual result in patients with POE is bacterial virulence level. Streptococcal strains are often virulent, producing exotoxins, and thus are associated with poor visual outcome.

20.2.5 Prophylaxis

Prophylaxis regimens against infectious POE differ in several countries.[24,25,26] In 2013, the ESCRS have published guidelines on prevention and treatment of POE.[15] Surgical procedures should be performed in specially prepared operating theaters (proper air-flow design, sterile and/or single-used equipment); washing hands with an antiseptic soap solution, mask, gowning, and sterile gloves are recommended. Topical povidone–iodine (PVI) should be used for antisepsis of the periocular skin area, cornea, and conjunctival sac. The 5 to 10% PVI solution should be left in place at the skin surface to act for at least 3 minutes. In case of any contraindications (allergy or hyperthyroidism), it can be replaced with the 0.05% solution of chlorhexidine. The surgical site should be scrupulously prepared and lids should be thoroughly draped to ensure adequate eyelash coverage. For conjunctiva and cornea antisepsis, 5% PVI solution should be left in the conjunctival sac for at least 3 minutes. It is important not to use PVI solution containing a detergent as it irreversibly coagulates the cornea. ESCRS guidelines also recommend applying 1-mg cefuroxime in 0.1-mL saline (0.9%) by intracameral injection at the end of surgery, as it has been proven that this maneuver reduces the POE rates by severalfold.[15] In 2012, specific commercial cefuroxime sodium at the necessary concentration (0.1 mg/mL) for intracameral use called Aprokam (Laboratories Théa, Clermont-Ferrand, France) received approval by the European Medicines Agency (EMA) and was introduced to the European market. By now, it is officially approved for intracameral antibiotic-prophylaxis of POE after cataract surgery in most European countries. Each vial contains 50 mg of cefuroxime to be reconstituted with 5 mL of saline solution and administered in the amount of 0.1 mL into the anterior chamber at the end of cataract surgery. Aprokam is a broad-spectrum antibiotic and covers most gram-positive and gram-negative organisms commonly associated with postoperative infectious endophthalmitis, including staphylococci, streptococci (except

Table 20.2 Pathogens causing postoperative endophthalmitis in different countries

Pathogens	Lundström et al,[11] Sweden	Friling et al,[7] Sweden	Mollan et al,[17] United Kingdom	Pijl et al,[18] The Netherlands	Han et al,[19] United States	Cheng et al,[20] Taiwan	Anand,[21] India	Kunimoto et al,[22] India	Sheng et al,[23] China
Gram-positive organisms	35%					44%	37.6%	53%	74%
Staphylococci									
Staphylococcus aureus			5%	12%	10%	24%	8%		12%
Coagulase-negative Staphylococcus		26%	62%	54%	70%	3%	13%	33%	46%
Enterococci	30%	31%	3%	2%	2%	12%	2%		7%
Other gram-positive organisms	13.5%	6%	3%	5%	3%	3%	11%		3%
Streptococci		7%	20%	19%	9%	3%	4%	10%	6%
Gram-negative organisms (*Pseudomonas* sp., *Enterobacteria* sp.)	12.5%	14%	7%	6%	6%	56%	41.7%	26%	13%
Negative cultures	16.5%	13%							
Fungi					–		21.8%	17%	13%
Actinomycete-related organisms								4%	

145

methicillin-resistant *S. aureus*, methicillin-resistant *S. epidermidis*, and *Enterococcus faecalis*), gram-negative bacteria (except *Pseudomonas aeruginosa*), and *P. acnes*. It is also important to treat properly preexisting infections, such as blepharitis, conjunctivitis, or dacryocystitis as well as infections in contralateral eye and socket.

The role of topical antibiotics in POE as preoperative prophylaxis is controversial and the regime differs in several countries.[27,28] It has been shown that the addition of topical antibiotics to PVI does not provide additional reduction in bacterial colonization of conjunctival sac.[27,28,29,30] ESCRS guidelines state that the use of topical antibiotics preoperatively and/or postoperatively does not have any specific benefit over the use of chlorhexidine or PVI preoperatively and over intracameral antibiotics injected at the close of surgery.[15] Although postoperative topical antibiotics are used in majority of European countries for 5 to 7 days, their preoperative use has declined in recent years. In Sweden and Denmark, most surgeons avoid using topical antibiotics before and after cataract surgery, as they are not recommended by national guidelines in standard cases. Topical antibiotics reduce selected sensitive conjunctival flora, unlike antiseptics, that is, PVI that reduces all conjunctival bacterial growth. Furthermore, topical PVI is the only intervention that has been demonstrated by a randomized clinical trial (RCT) to reduce the risk of POE.[31]

The choice of postoperative antisepsis should be at the surgeon's discretion, after evaluating the postoperative state of a patient and assessment of complications that occurred. In a noninflamed eye, the antibiotic weakly penetrates inside the globe; thus, intravenous antibiotic prophylaxis is not recommended. Oral antibiotic prophylaxis is recommend exclusively in cases of coexisting severe atopic disease, as the lid margins are more frequently colonized with *S. aureus*.

20.2.6 Treatment

The EVS, conducted in the early 1990s, is to date the only multicenter, prospective, RCT evaluating the roles of PPV and vitreous tap (VT) in the management of POE after cataract surgery. The EVS study concluded that vitrectomy is of substantial benefit for patients with initial visual acuity no better than light perception only.[16] However, more recent studies have shown that early vitrectomy is beneficial for patients with better visual acuity, as it immediately reduces the inflammatory debris in vitreous cavity, removes nontransparent medium allowing inspection of the retina, provides better access of intravitreally administered drugs to the tissues and also provides an adequate specimen for microbiological diagnosis (▶ Fig. 20.2). The decision to perform a surgery should always be driven by the clinical appearance and course. ESCRS guidelines on prevention, investigation, and management of POE (2013) consider an immediate PPV performed by a vitreoretinal surgeon as a gold standard of treatment of acute POE.[15] When a

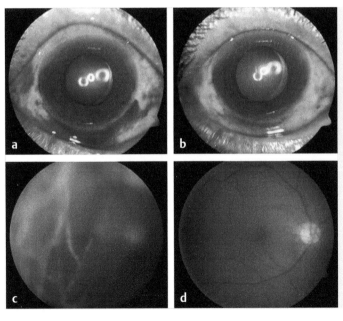

Fig. 20.2 Postoperative endophthalmitis resolution with pars plana vitrectomy. **(a)** Post cataract surgery, the patient presents with decreased vision and poor fundal glow on postoperative day 5. **(b)** Improved red fundal glow following pars plana vitrectomy (PPV). **(c)** Intraoperative image during PPV depicting cloudy vitreous with strands. **(d)** Completely resolved vitreous strands with good fundal glow following PPV.

vitreoretinal surgeon and a vitreoretinal operating room are not available immediately, the silver standard would be a vitreous biopsy with a vitreous cutter and not with a syringe and needle. Subsequently, antibiotics should be injected intravitreally and repeated as necessary according to the clinical response at intervals of 48 to 72 hours. Full vitrectomy should be considered later. It should be emphasized that EVS showed no harmful effect of vitrectomy compared with the VT; however, the study excluded the most severe cases of POE.

Samples of infected vitreous (▶ Fig. 20.2c) should always be collected for microbiology examination (gram stain, culture, or PCR), followed by intravitreal injection of antibiotics. First-choice therapy should be a combination of vancomycin 1 mg/0.1 mL and ceftazidime 2 mg/0.1 mL. Second choice is a combination of amikacin 400 μg/0.1 mL and vancomycin 2 mg/0.1 mL. Each drug should be injected from a separate syringe and a 30-gauge needle. At the same time, 400 μg of preservative-free dexamethasone should be injected into the vitreous. In the case of acute, virulent endophthalmitis, systemic therapy with the same antibiotics as those injected intravitreally should be applied for 48 hours. Moreover, systemic therapy with corticosteroids (prednisolone 1 or even 2 mg/kg/d) should be considered. For presumed fungal etiology, intravitreal injection of amphotericin B or voriconazole is recommended, without intravitreal steroids.

The EVS study showed no difference in final visual acuity or media clarity with or without systemic antibiotics.[16] As systemically administered antibiotics are not likely to provide additional benefit for treatment, omission of this kind of treatment may reduce toxic effects, costs (associated with their price and the costs of hospitalization required for intravenous drug administration), and length of hospital stay.[24] ESCRS guidelines recommended considering additional systemic antibiotic therapy with the same drugs used for intravitreal injections only in case of severe acute purulent endophthalmitis.

20.3 Toxic Anterior Segment Syndrome

TASS is an acute, sterile, postoperative inflammatory reaction in the anterior segment, caused by a noninfectious substance resulting in toxic damage to intraocular tissues. Its incidence is low (from 0.1 to 2%), and the mild cases usually recover spontaneously in a short period so they usually remain unnoticed and the serious cases are very rare. The process starts within days (typically 12–24 hours) after cataract surgery, and is responsive to topical steroids. Gram stains and culture results are always negative. It can occur as an isolated case; however, it usually presents as outbreaks. In some cases, it is hard to distinguish TASS from endophthalmitis because of similar clinical picture. In case of any doubt, the patient should be regarded as having infectious endophthalmitis and immediately treated. The most common symptoms of TASS are diffuse limbus-to-limbus corneal edema due to endothelial cell layer damage, fibrinous reaction in the anterior chamber, and hypopyon due to breakdown of the blood–aqueous barrier. In more severe cases, patients may present dilated, fixed, or irregular pupils, as well as increased intraocular pressure due to damage to the iris and trabecular meshwork. Patients usually report blurred vision and minimal or no pain. The distinguishing feature of TASS is absence of vitritis, as it is limited to the anterior segment, whereas endophthalmitis involves the posterior segment of the eye. ▶ Table 20.3 summarizes the

Table 20.3 Symptoms of toxic anterior segment syndrome versus infectious endophthalmitis

Characteristics	Toxic anterior segment syndrome	Infectious endophthalmitis
Onset	1–3 d	3–7 d
Symptoms	Usually no pain (or mild to moderate), blurred vision	Pain, significantly decreased visual acuity
Cornea	Significant edema (limbus-to-limbus) 2 to 3 +	Edema 1 to 2 +
Anterior chamber	Cells 1 to 3 +	Cells 3 +
	Fibrin 1 to 3 +	Fibrin variable
	Hypopyon 1 +	Hypopyon 3 +
Vitreous	Clear	Vitritis
Response to steroids	Positive	Negative

differentiating features between TASS and infectious endophthalmitis.

The causes of TASS are numerous and difficult to isolate. They can be categorized into three main groups: extraocular substances that unintentionally entered the anterior chamber during or after cataract surgery, substances introduced to the anterior chamber as a part of standard surgical procedure, or irritants on the surface of surgical devices that have accumulated due to inappropriate instrument cleaning and/or sterilization process. Review of the literature indicates that TASS can result from intraocular solutions with inappropriate chemical composition, concentration, pH, or osmolality, preservatives, denatured ophthalmic viscosurgical devices (OVDs), enzymatic detergents, heat-stable bacterial endotoxin from overgrowth of gram-negative bacilli in water baths of ultrasonic cleaners, oxidized metal deposits and residues, and factors related to IOLs such as residues from polishing or sterilizing compounds.[32] The box below presents the known causes of TASS.

> ### Known Causes of TASS (Adapted from Mamalis et al[32])
>
> - Irrigating solutions or OVDs:
>   - Incomplete chemical composition.
>   - Incorrect pH (< 6.5 or > 8.5).
>   - Incorrect osmolality (< 200 or > 400 mOsm)
>   - Preservatives or additives (e.g., antibiotics, dilating medications)
> - Ophthalmic instrument contaminants
>   - Detergent residues (ultrasonic, soaps, enzymatic cleaners)
>   - Bacterial lipopolysaccharides or other endotoxin residues
>   - Metal ion residues (copper and iron)
>   - Denatured OVDs
> - Ocular medications
>   - Incorrect drug concentration
>   - Incorrect pH (< 6.5 or > 8.5)
>   - Incorrect osmolality (< 200 or > 400 mOsm).
>   - Vehicle with wrong pH or osmolality.
>   - Preservatives in medication solution.
> - Intraocular lenses:
>   - Polishing compounds.
>   - Cleaning and sterilizing compounds.

The treatment of TASS involves intensive topical corticosteroids (in some cases accompanied with oral treatment) combined with cycloplegics. Most cases respond rapidly to topical steroids given every 30 to 60 minutes for the first 2 days with gradual tapering. It is advisable to perform gonioscopy, and monitor IOP as well as endothelial cell count.[15] Immediate anterior chamber washout is not recommended. Most of the cases clear within several days; however, more severe cases may experience long-term corneal edema necessitating a corneal transplant, or may result in intractable glaucoma and cystoid macular edema.

Every time, the outbreak of TASS requires thorough analysis of each surgical step and all possible risk factors, especially newly introduced medical substances and devices, its sterilization, storage, and transport conditions, to identify and eradicate the causative agent. In order to help trace the causes of TASS cases or outbreaks, the American Society of Cataract and Refractive Surgery (ASCRS) physician members and Ophthalmic Industry Partners have formed the ASCRS TASS task force that has launched a TASS-reporting questionnaire to record details of surgical procedures. This questionnaire is available at http://tassregistry.org/tass-combined-survey.cfm.

20.4 Vitritis

There are also various clinical conditions that present with vitritis and may mimic as infectious endophthalmitis. These conditions should be always differentiated from endophthalmitis; however, it is important to remember that concomitant endophthalmitis may also be present.

Retained lens fragments, exacerbation of preexisting uveitis, may cause sterile vitritis or it may be a symptom of injection-related sterile intraocular inflammation. Patients with retained lens material in the vitreous may develop intraocular inflammation (even with hypopyon) in the absence of infection and they also have an increased risk for endophthalmitis. If retained lens fragments are suspected, diagnostic ultrasound is particularly useful. Lens material usually appears as reflective, mobile material in the vitreous cavity; however, when involved with extensive epiretinal inflammatory membranes, it may not be mobile at the time of examination.

Exacerbation of preexisting uveitis after cataract surgery may also be accompanied with vitritis. Patients with a history of uveitis require adequate preoperative management, and proper control of inflammation before proceeding with intraocular surgery. As soon as endophthalmitis is ruled out, the patient should be treated with topical anti-inflammatory drugs and systemic corticosteroids or corticosteroid-sparing agents. Some cases of sterile inflammation after intravitreal injection of aflibercept were also described in the literature.[33],[34] Patients presented after intravitreal injection of aflibercept without pain, but with blurred vision, vitritis, and hazy view of the posterior segment. The visual outcomes were generally favorable in these cases.

Whenever a POE presents an ocular inflammatory response following cataract surgery, the ophthalmologist should suspect endophthalmitis and treat it as such with no delay, until proven otherwise. Proper and immediate treatment leads to optimal clinical results with recovery of useful vision.

20.5 Key Pearls

- Intraocular infections and inflammations are significant complications of cataract surgery limiting the visual potential of the eye, and even leading to blindness in severe cases.
- The role of topical antibiotics as a preoperative prophylaxis in POE is controversial as they do not have any specific benefit over the use of chlorhexidine or PVI preoperatively and intracameral antibiotics injected at the close of surgery.
- Whenever an ocular inflammatory response occurs after cataract surgery, endophthalmitis should be suspected and treated with no delay, until proven otherwise. Proper and immediate treatment leads to optimal clinical results with recovery of useful vision.
- The main treatment of POE is injection of intravitreal antibiotics preceded by either VT biopsy or vitrectomy. First-choice antibiotics are vancomycin (1 mg) and ceftazidime (2 mg).
- The outbreak of TASS requires thorough analysis of each surgical step and all possible risk factors (especially newly introduced medical substances and devices, its sterilization, storage, and transport conditions) to identify and eradicate the causative agent.

References

[1] Romero P, Méndez I, Salvat M, Fernández J, Almena M. Intracameral cefazolin as prophylaxis against endophthalmitis in cataract surgery. J Cataract Refract Surg. 2006; 32(3): 438–441

[2] Endophthalmitis Study Group, European Society of Cataract & Refractive Surgeons. Prophylaxis of postoperative endophthalmitis following cataract surgery: results of the ESCRS multicenter study and identification of risk factors. J Cataract Refract Surg. 2007; 33(6):978–988

[3] Yu-Wai-Man P, Morgan SJ, Hildreth AJ, Steel DH, Allen D. Efficacy of intracameral and subconjunctival cefuroxime in preventing endophthalmitis after cataract surgery. J Cataract Refract Surg. 2008; 34(3):447–451

[4] Garat M, Moser CL, Martín-Baranera M, Alonso-Tarrés C, Alvarez-Rubio L. Prophylactic intracameral cefazolin after cataract surgery: endophthalmitis risk reduction and safety results in a 6-year study. J Cataract Refract Surg. 2009; 35(4): 637–642

[5] García-Sáenz MC, Arias-Puente A, Rodríguez-Caravaca G, Bañuelos JB. Effectiveness of intracameral cefuroxime in preventing endophthalmitis after cataract surgery ten-year comparative study. J Cataract Refract Surg. 2010; 36(2):203–207

[6] Barreau G, Mounier M, Marin B, Adenis JP, Robert PY. Intracameral cefuroxime injection at the end of cataract surgery to reduce the incidence of endophthalmitis: French study. J Cataract Refract Surg. 2012; 38(8):1370–1375

[7] Friling E, Lundström M, Stenevi U, Montan P. Six-year incidence of endophthalmitis after cataract surgery: Swedish national study. J Cataract Refract Surg. 2013; 39(1):15–21

[8] Rodríguez-Caravaca G, García-Sáenz MC, Villar-Del-Campo MC, Andrés-Alba Y, Arias-Puente A. Incidence of endophthalmitis and impact of prophylaxis with cefuroxime on cataract surgery. J Cataract Refract Surg. 2013; 39(9):1399–1403

[9] Beselga D, Campos A, Castro M, et al. Postcataract surgery endophthalmitis after introduction of the ESCRS protocol: a 5-year study. Eur J Ophthalmol. 2014; 24(4):516–519

[10] Rahman N, Murphy CC. Impact of intracameral cefuroxime on the incidence of postoperative endophthalmitis following cataract surgery in Ireland. Ir J Med Sci. 2015; 184(2):395–398

[11] Lundström M, Friling E, Montan P. Risk factors for endophthalmitis after cataract surgery: predictors for causative organisms and visual outcomes. J Cataract Refract Surg. 2015; 41(11):2410–2416

[12] Creuzot-Garcher C, Benzenine E, Mariet AS, et al. Incidence of acute postoperative endophthalmitis after cataract surgery: a nationwide study in France from 2005 to 2014. Ophthalmology. 2016; 123(7):1414–1420

[13] Daien V, Papinaud L, Gillies MC, et al. Effectiveness and safety of an intracameral injection of cefuroxime for the prevention of endophthalmitis after cataract surgery with or without perioperative capsular rupture. JAMA Ophthalmol. 2016; 134 (7):810–816

[14] Lundström M, Barry P, Henry Y, Rosen P, Stenevi U. Evidence-based guidelines for cataract surgery: guidelines based on data in the European Registry of Quality Outcomes for Cataract and Refractive Surgery database. J Cataract Refract Surg. 2012; 38(6):1086–1093

[15] Barry P, Cordovés L, Gardner S. ESCRS guidelines on prevention and treatment of endophthalmitis following cataract surgery. European Society for Cataract and Refractive Surgeons; 2013. Available at: http://www.escrs.org/endophthalmitis/guidelines/ENGLISH.pdf

[16] Endophthalmitis Vitrectomy Study Group. Results of the endophthalmitis vitrectomy study. A randomized trial of immediate vitrectomy and of intravenous antibiotics for the treatment of postoperative bacterial endophthalmitis. Arch Ophthalmol. 1995; 113(12):1479–1496

[17] Mollan SP, Gao A, Lockwood A, Durrani OM, Butler L. Postcataract endophthalmitis: incidence and microbial isolates in a United Kingdom region from 1996 through 2004. J Cataract Refract Surg. 2007; 33(2):265–268

[18] Pijl BJ, Theelen T, Tilanus MA, Rentenaar R, Crama N. Acute endophthalmitis after cataract surgery: 250 consecutive

cases treated at a tertiary referral center in the Netherlands. Am J Ophthalmol. 2010; 149(3):482–7.e1, 2

[19] Han DP, Wisniewski SR, Wilson LA, et al. Spectrum and susceptibilities of microbiologic isolates in the endophthalmitis vitrectomy study. Am J Ophthalmol. 1996; 122(1):1–17

[20] Cheng JH, Chang YH, Chen CL, Chen YH, Lu DW, Chen JT. Acute endophthalmitis after cataract surgery at a referral centre in Northern Taiwan: review of the causative organisms, antibiotic susceptibility, and clinical features. Eye (Lond). 2010; 24(8):1359–1365

[21] Anand AR, Therese KL, Madhavan HN. Spectrum of aetiological agents of postoperative endophthalmitis and antibiotic susceptibility of bacterial isolates. Indian J Ophthalmol. 2000; 48(2):123–128

[22] Kunimoto DY, Das T, Sharma S, et al. Endophthalmitis Research Group. Microbiologic spectrum and susceptibility of isolates: part I. Postoperative endophthalmitis. Am J Ophthalmol. 1999; 128(2):240–242

[23] Sheng Y, Sun W, Gu Y, Lou J, Liu W. Endophthalmitis after cataract surgery in China, 1995–2009. J Cataract Refract Surg. 2011; 37(9):1715–1722

[24] Grzybowski A, Schwartz SG, Matsuura K, et al. Endophthalmitis prophylaxis in cataract surgery: overview of current practice patterns around the world. Curr Pharm Des. 2017; 23(4):565–573

[25] Schwartz SG, Grzybowski A, Flynn HW, Jr. Antibiotic prophylaxis: different practice patterns within and outside the United States. Clin Ophthalmol. 2016; 10:251–256

[26] Schwartz SG, Flynn HW, Jr, Grzybowski A, Relhan N, Ferris FL, III. Intracameral antibiotics and cataract surgery: endoph-thalmitis rates, costs, and stewardship. Ophthalmology. 2016; 123(7):1411–1413

[27] Shimada H, Nakashizuka H, Grzybowski A. Prevention and treatment of postoperative endophthalmitis using povidone-iodine. Curr Pharm Des. 2017; 23(4):574–585

[28] Kuklo P, Grzybowski A, Schwartz SG, Flynn HW, Pathengay A. Hot topics in perioperative antibiotics for cataract surgery. Curr Pharm Des. 2017; 23(4):551–557

[29] Grzybowski A, Kukło P, Pieczyński J, Beiko G. A review of preoperative manoeuvres for prophylaxis of endophthalmitis in intraocular surgery: topical application of antibiotics, disinfectants, or both? Curr Opin Ophthalmol. 2016; 27(1):9–23

[30] Grzybowski A. Controversial role of topical antibiotics in endophthalmitis prophylaxis for cataract surgery. JAMA Ophthalmol. 2015; 133(4):490–491

[31] Ciulla TA, Starr MB, Masket S. Bacterial endophthalmitis prophylaxis for cataract surgery: an evidence-based update. Ophthalmology. 2002; 109(1):13–24

[32] Mamalis N, Edelhauser HF, Dawson DG, Chew J, LeBoyer RM, Werner L. Toxic anterior segment syndrome. J Cataract Refract Surg. 2006; 32(2):324–333

[33] Grewal DS, Schwartz T, Fekrat S. Sequential sterile intraocular inflammation associated with consecutive intravitreal injections of aflibercept and ranibizumab. Ophthalmic Surg Lasers Imaging Retina. 2017; 48(5):428–431

[34] Kim JY, You YS, Kwon OW, Kim SH. Sterile inflammation after intravitreal injection of aflibercept in a Korean population. Korean J Ophthalmol. 2015; 29(5):325–330

21 Intraoperative Aberrometry

Kathryn M. Hatch

Abstract

Intraoperative aberrometry (IA) is a proven technology to optimize refractive outcomes in cataract surgery. Given the increasing patient expectation for optimal refractive outcomes after cataract surgery, IA may provide significant value for a variety of clinical scenarios. It is used for spherical intraocular lens (IOL) power calculation for normal eyes and may have a unique role for extreme axial lengths (< 22.5 and > 26.5 mm). Additionally, it has been shown to assist in maximizing outcomes with astigmatism management including toric IOLs and limbal relaxing incisions (LRIs). During toric IOL surgery, both the spherical and toric powers are selected in the aphakic state, followed by axis alignment optimization in the pseudophakic state. Both the anterior and posterior contribution to the eye's cylinder is accounted for as light is projected onto the retina, and the reflected images pass through the optical system of the eye. Femtosecond laser-assisted arcuate incisions as well as manual LRIs can also be optimized with IA. Additionally, IA may play a crucial role in the postrefractive eye in optimizing residual refractive errors. This could ultimately lead to less postoperative excimer enhancements or the need for IOL exchange or piggyback IOLs. The technology does have potential limitations including cost and additional operating room time. Additionally, the readings are sensitive to intracameral bubbles, intraocular pressure, or pressure from the lid speculum, so there is a user learning curve to the device.

Keywords: intraoperative aberrometry, refractive cataract surgery, optimization cataract surgery, residual refractive error

21.1 Introduction

Intraoperative aberrometry (IA) is a promising technology that aids in optimizing refractive outcomes for cataract surgery. In the era of increasing patient demands for spectacle independence, achieving targeted refractive outcomes is essential to patient satisfaction. Efforts to improve intraocular lens (IOL) outcomes have traditionally focused on optimizing preoperative biometry measurements and IOL power prediction formulas. But even with the most advanced preoperative calculations including noncontact biometry, averages of

multiple corneal power measurements, and optimization of a surgeon-specific A-constant for each IOL, it is still not uncommon to have suboptimal refractive results. Even among the most experienced surgeons, only 80% of eyes are within of ±0.50 diopters of intended spherical target.[1] Larger deviations from intended target are routinely seen in high myopes,[2] high hyperopes, eyes that have undergone prior corneal refractive surgery,[3,4] and eyes in which it is impossible to obtain biometry, such as a white or dense posterior subcapsular cataract.

IA takes real-time phakic, aphakic, and pseudophakic refractions during cataract surgery. The aphakic refraction provides both a spherical and toric power calculation for optimal IOL power selection. In cases of toric IOL implantation, in additional to the IOL power selection, the optimal axis alignment can be obtained in the pseudophakic state with real-time feedback from the aberrometer to guide fine-tune axis alignment. It can also be used to titrate limbal relaxing incision (LRI) and may have a key role in IOL selection in the postrefractive patient.

The first commercially available intraoperative wavefront aberrometer was the ORange (WaveTec Vision), which was later updated to the Optiwave Refractive Analysis (ORA) system (Alcon) in July 2013. Light is projected onto the retina, and the reflected images pass through the optical system of the eye, distorting its wavefront, which is subsequently analyzed according to optical and mathematical principles proprietary to the device. The ORA uses a super luminescent light-emitting diode and Talbot–Moiré interferometer, where the wavefront passes through gratings set at specific distances producing a specific fringe pattern, taking 40 measurements within seconds, while combining data obtained from the central 4-mm optical zone. Aberrations in the wavefront cause distortions in the fringe pattern, which translates to a refractive value using proprietary algorithms, and ultimately determines spherical, cylindrical, and axis components of the refractive error.[5,6,7] The ORA takes into account parameters such as posterior corneal astigmatism and higher-order aberrations, allowing the surgeon to confirm or revise the IOL power chosen according to traditional preoperative biometry or with online calculators for toric IOLs.[5,6] The advantages of this system are that it is compact and lightweight (allowing easy attachment to the microscope) and can be configured to have a dynamic range of –5.0 to +20 diopters without degradation of the fringe pattern.

21.2 IOL Optimization and Normal and Extreme Axial Lengths

Each IOL model goes through a lens optimization process with ORA. Initially, a global set of regression coefficients and manufacturer lens constant is assigned after the following parameters:

- ≥ 100 surgeries with at least 10 days of postoperative data.
- ≥ 3 surgeons with ≥ 15 surgeries.
- No surgeon with greater than 50% of surgeries performed.

Once a surgeon has greater than 25 cases with good data, the surgeon-specific optimization can be done and the surgeon-specific IOL constant can be applied. The gold and platinum bars seen on the IOL screen page designate if the IOL has global or surgeon-specific lens optimization (▶ Fig. 21.1).

The use of IA in routine cataract surgery is not well defined. Given that there are variables that can affect the reading including pressure from the eyelid speculum, patient fixation, as well as the

intraocular pressure (IOP) or intracameral bubbles, a surgeon learning curve or intra-user error can affect readings. A study by Davison et al showed that IA in eyes with no prior eye surgery did not improve overall clinical outcomes, but it may be helpful when there is a significant difference between IA and preoperative calculations.[8]

IA for axial myopia and short eyes may also have a role. For axial myopes, defined at axial length greater than 25 mm, when compared to preoperative biometry using Sanders–Retzlaff–Kraff (SRK)/T, Holladay 1 and 2, Barrett Universal II, and Hill-RBF, IA was shown to be better than all formulas and was as effective as the axial length–optimized Holladay 1 formula in predicting residual refractive error and reducing hyperopic outcomes.[9] Extreme axial lengths, including short eyes less than 22.5 mm and long eyes greater than 26.5 mm, are also good candidates for maximizing refractive outcomes with aberrometry. Prediction errors have been reduced by software updates that optimize lens coefficients by axial length group.

21.3 Astigmatism Management

21.3.1 Toric Intraocular Lens

As astigmatism correction with toric IOLs and LRIs at the time of cataract surgery has become more

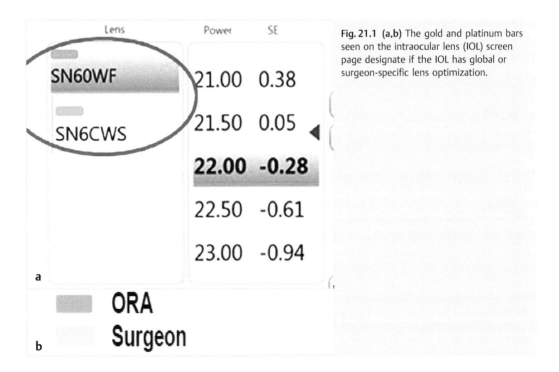

Fig. 21.1 (a,b) The gold and platinum bars seen on the intraocular lens (IOL) screen page designate if the IOL has global or surgeon-specific lens optimization.

mainstream, and as patient expectations for uncorrected visual acuity after surgery have risen, increased accuracy is also expected. IA assists not only with spherical and toric IOL power in the aphakic state, but also with IOL rotation and ideal axis determination in the pseudophakic state. At the time of surgery, generally patients are marked preoperatively by the surgeon while seated in an upright position using a three-pronged marker to reference axis marks at the corneal limbus. The steep axis can be marked with small femtosecond laser-assisted arcuate incisions (FSAIs) or manually under the operating microscope. During surgery, IA is used initially to obtain an aphakic reading to determine spherical and toric power selection. After the power is chosen and IOL implanted, the reticule function can be turned on to guide initial gross alignment and then subsequent fine-tuning of axis placement. Once the IOL is grossly aligned, pseudophakic refraction is performed while the patient is fixated on a target light to assist with final axis alignment. Prior to this reading, viscoelastic material is removed, the eye is pressurized and a reading is taken, and one of the following recommendations is provided: clockwise, counterclockwise, or NRR (no rotation required). If clockwise or counterclockwise is encountered, the surgeon can opt to reposition the IOL. Pseudophakic rotations, if required, can be repeated with IA measurements until it was decided that astigmatism had been optimally minimized in the surgeon's judgment. In a small series in a private practice setting, it was found that with the use of IA, postoperative residual refractive astigmatism of ≤ 0.50 diopters

was 2.5 times more likely with the use of the ORA compared with standard techniques.[10]

21.3.2 Limbal Relaxing Incisions

LRI management can be done and titrated in the phakic, aphakic, and pseudophakic states. Typically, a reading is obtained prior to or after manual LRIs or after FSAIs, most often in the aphakic state just before IOL implantation, and power of the cylinder (D) and axis is provided. The surgeon can then titrate the LRIs based on the readings. Anterior penetrating FSAIs can be opened to augment the effect or could be elongated with a blade in an attempt to achieve less than 0.5 diopters of astigmatism.

In eyes with prior laser in situ keratomileusis (LASIK) flaps, IA-guided manual LRIs can be formed to reduce astigmatism in this postrefractive group. FSAIs are often avoided in eyes with prior LASIK to prevent disruption of the LASIK flap. Another situation that an IA-guided manual LRI might be considered is in eyes that have ≤ 0.5 diopters on preoperative testing when it is not clear whether the patient needs any astigmatism correction at the time of cataract surgery. In these cases, axis as well as posterior corneal astigmatism contribution to overall cylinder is determined and a manual LRI is made as needed based on ORA to achieve ≤ 0.5 diopter cylinder. When taking aphakic power calculation readings, the surgeon can also make a judgment as to whether additional LRI augmentation needs to be performed. ▶ Fig. 21.2 shows screenshots where no further LRI augmentation is required as there is ≤ 0.5 diopter cylinder as seen in

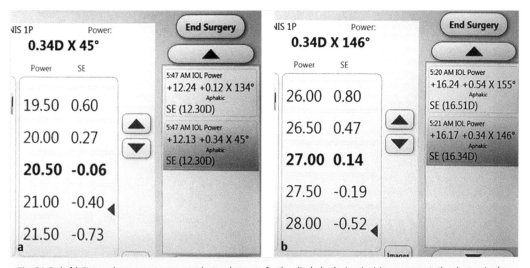

Fig. 21.2 **(a,b)** Figure demonstrates screenshots where no further limbal relaxing incision augmentation is required as there is ≤ 0.5 diopter cylinder as seen in the aphakic refraction.

the aphakic refraction. Additional LRI-specific readings can also be made with the IA for confirmation. In a retrospective study by Packer,[6] the use of IA to guide LRI enhancements reduced the frequency of subsequent excimer laser enhancement to treat residual cylinder compared to eyes in which IA was not used.

21.3.3 Prior Refractive Surgery

Achieving the refractive target for eyes having undergone refractive surgery including LASIK, phototherapeutic keratectomy (PRK), and radial keratotomy (RK) poses particular challenges when attempting to obtain a desired refractive outcome. Additionally, this population is by nature more demanding of their refractive outcomes given that they have previously undergone a spectacle-sparing procedure. Using traditionally measured average keratometry values taken in the office fails to accurately measure the anterior corneal curvature in these eyes and, if used, would result in a hyperopic refractive surprise.[11] Correction factors have been used to reduce these refractive surprises in postrefractive surgery eyes. In a series of 173 eyes, McCarthy et al found that more than 45% of postrefractive surgery eyes fell outside ±0.50 diopters of the intended target refraction, despite adjustments to traditional formulas.[12]

Given these measurement challenges, IA may be an aid in improving refractive results and may reduce the postoperative enhancement rate. Ianchulev et al[4] showed the advantage of IA compared to standard biometry in a series of eyes with prior LASIK or PRK correction, demonstrating a statistically significant increase in the accuracy of predicted manifest refraction spherical equivalent with aberrometry compared to the Haigis L, Shammas, and combination of all clinical data based on surgeon's choice.

21.3.4 Unique Situations

IA can be used in specific situations to manage refractive surprises or residual refractive astigmatism after cataract surgery. In the case of piggyback IOL, a pseudophakic reading can be obtained after cataract surgery and the piggyback IOL can be chosen based on the IA measurement (1.5 × spherical equivalent for hyperopic corrections and 1.2 × spherical equivalent for myopic corrections). Additionally, when postoperative residual refractive astigmatism with toric IOL is encountered due to malposition of the IOL, IA can

assist with ideal alignment. The LRI function can also be used in any state to minimize refractive astigmatism in these eyes.

21.4 Challenges with Aberrometry

IA readings must be taken in a standardized fashion to obtain the best-quality readings. Before capturing the readings, IOP must be adjusted using applanation tonometry after inflating the eye with either 0.9% balanced salt solution (BSS) or sodium hyaluronate 1% for the aphakic refraction or BSS for the pseudophakic refraction. The surgeon must ensure uniformity of the media in the anterior chamber as a mixture of materials, including retained dispersive viscoelastic or intracameral bubbles, can have significant effect on the accuracy of the readings. Additionally, prior to IA readings, care must be taken to ensure that the ocular surface was uniformly hydrated, and IOP is in the recommended range of 15 to 21 mm Hg measured with a Barraquer Tonometer (Ocular Instruments Inc., Bellevue, WA). The surgeon must ensure no distortion from the eyelid speculum was present. Other drawbacks of IA include cost (additional personnel and equipment required, out-of-pocket costs to the patient) and additional time in the operating room. There is also a learning curve for the surgeon, as certain variables mentioned earlier can affect results during use.

21.5 Conclusion

IA provides an additional resource in cataract surgery that can assist with refractive optimization and improved outcomes. IA can assist with many situations including spherical power calculations in normal and extreme axial lengths, astigmatism management with toric power selection and axis alignment and LRIs, as well as postrefractive eyes. IOL optimization and mastery of use with the device are necessary to provide best possible results.

21.6 Key Pearls

- IA is a promising technology that aids in optimizing refractive outcomes for cataract surgery.
- IA can be applied for astigmatism management in the cataract patient to minimize residual refractive cylinder for toric IOL and can be used to titrate LRIs.

- IA can assist with minimizing residual refractive errors in the postrefractive patient and may also have significant benefit for extreme axial lengths.
- IA can be used in unique refractive situations after cataract surgery including piggyback IOL selection and toric IOL rotation in the setting of refractive surprise and residual refractive astigmatism from toric IOL malposition, respectively.
- IOL optimization and mastery of use of IA are necessary for optimal outcomes.

References

[1] Hahn U, Krummenauer F, Kölbl B, et al. Determination of valid benchmarks for outcome indicators in cataract surgery: a multicenter, prospective cohort trial. Ophthalmology. 2011; 118(11):2105–2112

[2] Ghanem AA, El-Sayed HM. Accuracy of intraocular lens power calculation in high myopia. Oman J Ophthalmol. 2010; 3(3):126–130

[3] Canto AP, Chhadva P, Cabot F, et al. Comparison of IOL power calculation methods and intraoperative wavefront aberrometer in eyes after refractive surgery. J Refract Surg. 2013; 29 (7):484–489

[4] Ianchulev T, Hoffer KJ, Yoo SH, et al. Intraoperative refractive biometry for predicting intraocular lens power calculation after prior myopic refractive surgery. Ophthalmology. 2014; 121(1):56–60

[5] Wiley WF, Bafna S. Intra-operative aberrometry guided cataract surgery. Int Ophthalmol Clin. 2011; 51(2):119–129

[6] Packer M. Effect of intraoperative aberrometry on the rate of postoperative enhancement: retrospective study. J Cataract Refract Surg. 2010; 36(5):747–755

[7] Hemmati HD, Gologorsky D, Pineda R, II. Intraoperative wavefront aberrometry in cataract surgery. Semin Ophthalmol. 2012; 27(5–6):100–106

[8] Davison JA, Potvin R. Preoperative measurement vs intraoperative aberrometry for the selection of intraocular lens sphere power in normal eyes. Clin Ophthalmol. 2017; 11 (11):923–929

[9] Hill DC, Sudhakar S, Hill CS, et al. Intraoperative aberrometry versus preoperative biometry for intraocular lens power selection in axial myopia. J Cataract Refract Surg. 2017; 43 (4):505–510

[10] Hatch KM, Woodcock EC, Talamo JH. Intraocular lens power selection and positioning with and without intraoperative aberrometry. J Refract Surg. 2015; 31(4):237–242

[11] Seitz B, Langenbucher A. Intraocular lens power calculation in eyes after corneal refractive surgery. J Refract Surg. 2000; 16(3):349–361

[12] McCarthy M, Gavanski GM, Paton KE, Holland SP. Intraocular lens power calculations after myopic laser refractive surgery: a comparison of methods in 173 eyes. Ophthalmology. 2011; 118(5):940–944

22 Futuristic Approach and Advancements

Gary Wörtz

Abstract

Futuristic approach and advancements in cataract surgery provides a summary of the key features that will be changing over the next 10 to 20 years. This chapter discusses these advancements within the context of current unmet needs in the developed markets. The most important consideration is the current manpower shortage of cataract surgeons, which will be getting worse as the global population continues to age. Ophthalmologists will need to adapt processes and systems to improve their surgical efficiency and productivity while relying on optometrists and other providers to perform more of the pre- and postoperative care. Additionally, technology will need to become faster, easier to use, and more multifunctional to improve patient throughput. The second major unmet need is our ability to achieve the desired refractive results and to modify them postoperatively. Lens and laser technology are being developed that will allow for postoperative adjustment of optical style and power through less invasive and even noninvasive means. The third unmet need is the more complete correction of presbyopia, which would likely drive more patients to correct lens-based pathology earlier in their life. Finally, the idea of pharmaceutical treatment to prevent and reverse cataracts is discussed. All of these unmet needs require surgeons to adapt more efficient processes while partnering with industry to bring new technology to market.

Keywords: cataract, future lens implant, laser, ergonomics, presbyopia, management, light adjustable IOL, LAL

22.1 The Future Efficiency Centric Cataract Models

With an aging demographic in most countries, the need for cataract surgery is expected to continue accelerating, putting more pressure on the available surgeons to become increasingly efficient and productive to keep pace with demand. This will require cataract surgeons to spend the vast majority of their time in the operating room (OR), and further rely upon the division of labor model. Optometrists and other providers will be relied upon for most of the preoperative diagnosis, care, and counseling. Diagnostic equipment will need to become more useful, user independent, and efficient. With one simple scan, the patient's visual acuity, refraction, topography, biometric measurements, anterior segment and retinal images, as well as optical coherence tomography (OCT) of the macula and optic nerve will be obtained. Once there is the ability to change the power and refractive properties of the lens through noninvasive means postoperatively, biometric measurement, predictive formulas, and refractive targets will become less important. This advancement will clear the way for immediate sequential bilateral cataract surgery to become the new standard since there will be less need to learn from the refractive results of the first eye before operating on the second eye.[1]

The postoperative course will be typically managed by optometrists and eventually the refractive outcome will be finalized approximately 1 month after surgery through a laser or ultraviolet (UV) treatment to the lens, allowing patients to routinely achieve visual outcomes that were previously almost impossible. Patients will be able to preview their various visual outcomes (monovision, extended depth of focus, multifocality) using virtual reality in the office, and a lock-in procedure will give patients exactly what they want with a new level of precision and accuracy.

22.2 Preoperative Technology Advancements

In any modern ophthalmic office, there is typically at least one full room of individual pieces of equipment dedicated to gathering a portion of necessary data. Each device requires entry of patient data, patient positioning, patient cooperation and participation, and technician time and expertise, and takes up precious space. The model of single function equipment will need to adapt to the present and coming challenges to decrease time for patient throughput. Multifunctional equipment that can obtain all necessary measurements for a cataract surgery workup will need to quickly come of age. Already, there are biometers that combine OCT or laser interferometry and topography. There are topographers that incorporate autorefractor/autokeratometer and wavefront aberrometer functions.

OCTs incorporate fundus camera functions. The practice of the future will need to have access to equipment that places all of these functions within a single device or small suite of devices.

Another unmet need within the space of the preoperative assessment is in the realm of patient education. Great videos already exist that explain the risks, benefits, alternatives, and various options in cataract surgery. However, many patients arrive for their appointment unprepared to make the necessary decisions regarding their choice of lens technology. Many patients are hearing about the differences between near, intermediate, and distance vision for the first time and the stress of the requisite financial implications can make these choices harder. Given advancements in the field of virtual reality, it is now possible for patients to experience various visual scenarios in much more experiential ways. A virtual reality vision preview program will be essential to help patients make more informed decisions before surgery, and especially after surgery once lens technology like RxSight and Perfect lens come to market. Others have approached these decisions by utilizing technology to assess the visual needs of the patient in their normal environment. Surgiorithm and other companies are currently trying to tackle this problem by both photodocumenting vision-related activities and prompting the patient through a questionnaire.

22.3 Advances in the Operating Room

The OR equipment and organization will also be targets for innovation. To stay viable, technology will need to become smaller, more efficient, and more cost effective. It is likely that at some point, ultrasound phacoemulsification will become replaced with a new technology. One simple device that is challenging the current paradigm is the miLoop from Iantech. This device is a wire made from the shape memory metal, nitinol. Essentially, the miLoop is a retractable wire snare that when fully extended forms the shape of a cross section of a cataract, and naturally finds its way around the cortex to the poles of the nucleus. When the loop is retracted, it sections the lens into fragments. This quick maneuver can save time and potentially reduce ultrasound energy, saving endothelial cells in the process. This is a technology with a great deal of promise given its simplicity and effectiveness, especially for dense cataracts.

Additionally, femtosecond laser technology will need to advance and become more efficient and cost effective. The author predicts that the majority of femtosecond lasers will eventually migrate into the OR. Downward pressure on costs for using the laser will hopefully result in a scenario where surgeons can utilize the benefits of femtosecond laser technology on all their cataract cases.

Surgical ergonomics provide another area of unmet needs in the OR. Many studies have shown that approximately 50% of ophthalmologists suffer from back and neck pain at some point in their career and many have to limit their work due to the discomfort and disability it causes. Currently, ophthalmologists face a relatively high risk for cervical disc injury due to the poor ergonomics required for operating through a microscope. Added to that are the inconsistent positions of the bed height and foot pedals, making for a multifactorial equation. If operating temporally, staff must physically move the foot pedals when changing from right to left eyes or vice versa. Phacoemulsification units, microscopes, and beds all take up a significant footprint with significant wasted space surrounding each piece of equipment. To address these issues, a surgical cockpit will need to be developed that will allow surgeons to set the seat position, incline, and support to their individual needs. It will have attached foot pedals that can also be adjusted and set to preference. Just like a luxury car, each surgeon will be able to set his or her preference and have consistent ergonomic support. This seat will be attached to a track on the floor allowing surgeons to automatically change positions without any foot pedal or cord manipulation. The patient bed will also be connected to this system, and may automatically adjust to the desired height. The unused space under the bed may be utilized by other technology as well. Microscopes will likely be replaced by better and better 3D viewing systems that allow surgeons to operate in a much more comfortable position, which will increase their health, productivity, and longevity. Companies such as TrueVision have brought this advanced technology to market and it will undoubtedly continue to improve.

22.4 Lens Technology

In the next few years, the function of an IOL may change dramatically. Currently, surgeons and patients must agree on a style of lens and target for postoperative refraction. With few exceptions, if the result is off target or the patient does not

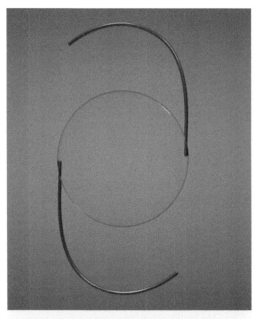

Fig. 22.1 Photosensitive three-piece silicon intraocular lens employed for light-adjustable therapy. (This image is provided courtesy of RxSight.)

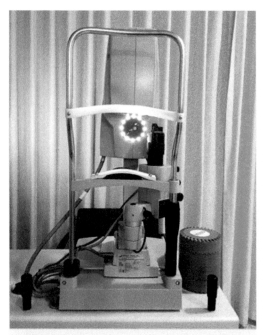

Fig. 22.2 Light delivery device that delivers ultraviolet-A light at 365-nm wavelength to the photosensitive silicon intraocular lens. (This image is provided courtesy of Kevin Miller.)

tolerate optical side effects of the technology, the lens must be exchanged or corneal refractive surgery performed. However, there are four categories of new technologies on the horizon that may be able to change that equation.[2]

The first technology is the light adjustable lens (▶ Fig. 22.1) from Rx Sight, formerly Calhoun Vision, which involves the use of a digital UV light source to cause photo polymerization of UV-sensitive macromeres within the optic.[3,4] Studies have shown incredible precision for treating myopia, hyperopia, as well as cylinder with long-term stability (▶ Fig. 22.2, ▶ Fig. 22.3, ▶ Fig. 22.4).

The second technology is from Perfect Lens. Their technology involves a femtosecond laser application to lenses in vivo that causes a change in refractive index.[5,6] This change creates a predictable and reversible change in the lens power, and can create and/or reverse toric or multifocal changes to IOLs. It has shown to be effective in acrylic lens types by altering the relative hydrophilicity of the material.

The third category of new IOL technology can be broadly defined as multicomponent IOLs represented by Infinite Vision Optics, ClarVista, and Omega Ophthalmics.[7] These lenses all have an element of modularity, allowing the addition or subtraction of optics (or other technology) without the removal of the haptics or body of the device. All of these technologies produce an easier way to exchange technology compared to the current standard. However, the Omega Gemini Refractive Capsule has the additional benefit of creating a protected environment within the natural capsule. As we know, the capsular bag is perhaps the most inert space within the eye and has safely held more medical implants than any other anatomical structure in the human history. The Omega device keeps this inert space open with the ambition to provide a platform for the safe housing of additional technology such as lenses, intraocular pressure sensors, as well as time-released drugs and drug delivery devices. This platform is agnostic to the type of add-on technology so long as it is also biologically inert and fits within the cavity created.

The fourth category of technology is the truly accommodative lens. We have seen great excitement in this category for decades, but have nevertheless seen little progress, with only one Food and Drug Administration (FDA) approved platform

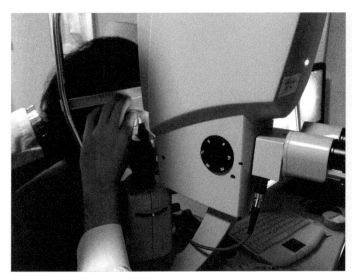

Fig. 22.3 Ultraviolet-A light being delivered to the light adjustable lens from RxSight. (This image is provided courtesy of Kevin Miller.)

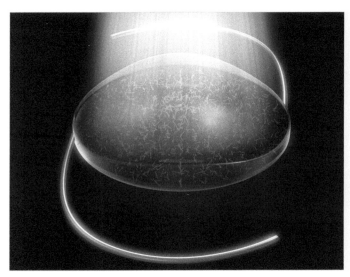

Fig. 22.4 The intraocular lens (IOL) is locked at its current refractive state, preventing any further change in the refractive status of the IOL. (This image is provided courtesy of RxSight.)

available. While research and development efforts to find a natural solution to couple ciliary muscle contraction with pseudophakic accommodation continue throughout the world, others have developed an exciting alternative approach using electronics. Elenza, along with Google and Alcon, have all taken steps to produce an electronic accommodating IOL using LCD technology with pupil sensors. Basically, the lens senses pupil constriction as a proxy for accommodation and provides an increase in the power of the lens. As with any electronic device, it requires a power source, which in this case is a battery. It is also not foldable and has a relatively small optical zone. Regardless of the

challenges, this is a robust technology that could truly change the game for patients and surgeons alike. Having a solution for presbyopia that will compete with a 20- or 30-year-old phakic lens could push demand for lens-based surgery into the mid-40 s as a routine procedure.

22.5 Prevention

A potential disruptive innovation in cataract surgery is a pharmaceutical treatment that prevents or reverses cataractous formation in the lens. In 2015, a study was published in Nature that showed great promise for the compound lanosterol that can prevent and reverse lens protein aggregation in both in vitro and in vivo animal models.[8] By preventing or reversing cataract formation, the field of cataract surgery could become almost entirely obsolete. If that situation arises, anterior segment surgeons would likely shift their focus to refractive surgery, which would have a stronger value proposition. The challenge faced by a pharmaceutical treatment for prevention of cataract surgery is largely financial. A monthly eye drop or injection will likely never be able to compete with the low cost of a one-time cataract surgery. The economic challenges of this, given the ubiquitous nature of cataracts, may be insurmountable despite its potential efficacy.

22.6 Key Pearls

- Future lens technology will be modular, modifiable, and exchangeable opening a new paradigm for achieving the desired refractive results.
- Once a lens implant is developed that can fully correct presbyopia without the optical trade-offs of multifocality, the age for lens replacement surgery will shift into the mid-40 s and mid-50 s.
- The demand for cataract surgery will continue to put pressure on surgeons to adapt processes and technology to improve efficiency and extend the productive years of each surgeon.
- The comanagement model of shared care between surgeons and optometrists will continue to evolve, allowing both providers to function in collaborative roles.

- Technology will need to continue advancing, by being developed with multiple functions, more user independent, and smaller in footprint.

Videos

Video 22.1 Demonstration of the mechanism of action of light-adjustable intraocular lens. (Used with permission of Rx Sight.)

References

[1] Singh R, Dohlman TH, Sun G. Immediately sequential bilateral cataract surgery: advantages and disadvantages. Curr Opin Ophthalmol. 2017; 28(1):81–86

[2] Wortz GN, Wortz PR. Refractive IOL Pipeline: Innovations, Predictions, and Needs. Curr Ophthalmol Rep. 2017; 5(3): 255–263

[3] Brierley L. Refractive results after implantation of a light-adjustable intraocular lens in postrefractive surgery cataract patients. Ophthalmology. 2013; 120(10):1968–1972

[4] Hengerer FH, Dick HB, Conrad-Hengerer I. Clinical evaluation of an ultraviolet light adjustable intraocular lens implanted after cataract removal: eighteen months follow-up. Ophthalmology. 2011; 118(12):2382–2388

[5] Bille JF, Engelhardt J, Volpp H-R, et al. Chemical basis for alteration of an intraocular lens using a femtosecond laser. Biomed Opt Express. 2017; 8(3):1390–1404

[6] Ford J, Werner L, Mamalis N. Adjustable intraocular lens power technology. J Cataract Refract Surg. 2014; 40(7): 1205–1223

[7] Portaliou DM, Grentzelos MA, Pallikaris IG. Multicomponent intraocular lens implantation: two-year follow-up. J Cataract Refract Surg. 2013; 39(4):578–584

[8] Zhao L, Chen XJ, Zhu J, et al. Lanosterol reverses protein aggregation in cataracts. Nature. 2015; 523(7562):607–611

23 Telescopic Intraocular Lenses

Isaac Lipshitz and Amar Agarwal

Abstract

The telescopic intraocular lenses (IOL) are specifically helpful in cases with macular degeneration. The telescopic IOL magnifies the image on the central retina, while the peripheral field remains normal. Hence, the IOL helps patients with central visual impairment as in macular degeneration to see the objects clearly.

Keywords: telescopic IOL, macular degeneration, AMD, dry AMD, wet AMD, central vision loss

23.1 Introduction

With an aging population and with the increased longevity that modern medicine has made possible, there is an increasing population of cataract patients with other associated eye diseases such as age-related macular degeneration (AMD), diabetes, etc., thus presenting to the eye surgeon with a complex situation. The difficulties that comorbid pathologies induce are being experienced by surgeons all over the world. The prevalence of AMD in Asia has been found to be similar to that in Caucasian populations and has been variously reported as ranging from 1.4 to 12.7% for early AMD and 0.2 to 1.9% for late AMD. The presence of cortical cataract and prior cataract surgery are significantly associated with increased prevalence of AMD, showing that these age-related conditions often coexist.

Dry AMD constitutes 85 to 90% of AMD patients and most of these patients have no medical treatment at all, other than vitamins and antioxidants. These patients can be treated only with optical means. Among the wet ARMD, only 10 to 15% can be assisted by medical treatment and these go on to become the dry types, who then again need to be visually rehabilitated. The important factor to realize here is that despite performing cataract surgery[1,2] successfully in these patients, they do not benefit as much visually because of the coexisting retinal pathology. There is, therefore, a significant difference between treating the disease pathology with medical management/lasers/cataract surgery and with being able to successfully rehabilitate the patient visually. Visual benefits from treatment are after all what actually affects the quality of life of the patient and what is meaningful to the patient.

23.2 A New Sulcus Implanted Mirror Telescopic IOL for Age-Related Macular Diseases and Other Macular Disorders the LMI-SI (OriLens)

Cataract surgery per se is not a problem in eyes with AMD, but lack of post-op visual improvement is definitely a cause of concern. One of us (Dr. Isaac Lipshitz) designed the LMI-SI (OriLens), which is a telescopic lens working on the principle of using mirrors to magnify the central image while the peripheral field remains normal. The LMI is designed in such a way that it is positioned in the sulcus over a regular bag implanted IOL. It is a telescopic IOL that is designed to magnify the image on the central retina. It looks like a regular polymethyl methacrylate (PMMA) IOL and is 5.00 to 6.00 mm in diameter (loop diameter is 13.50 mm), and it contains loops that have a similar configuration as a regular IOL. The only significant difference compared to a regular IOL is its central thickness. The LMI is thicker (central thickness of 1.25 mm, which is higher thickness than a normal IOL). The first worldwide implantation of this lens was done by Prof. Amar Agarwal.

23.3 Preoperative Evaluation

Preoperatively, as soon as a patient with AMD comes, a full medical eye examination including slit lamp for evaluation of the cornea, iris, anterior chamber, lens, and vitreous is done. A thorough retinal examination is done including fundus fluorescein angiography and optical coherence tomography, and the IOP is checked. The distance and near visual acuity are checked in each eye separately using the Early Treatment Diabetic Retinopathy Study (ETDRS) chart with best correction. The best corrected, distance, and near visual acuity with ×2.5 external telescope is again checked using the ETDRS chart. If a patient shows improvement with the external telescope, he or she is a good candidate for the LMI-SI (OriLens). A cycloplegic refraction is also done. Specular microscopy is done for endothelial cell count. A-scan is done for anterior chamber depth and IOL calculations. Keratometric readings are taken with the keratometer or with corneal topography.

23.4 Surgery for Implanting the LMI-SI (OriLens)

Intraoperatively, anesthesia is given according to the surgeon's preference. A corneal or limbal incision may be used and the size of the incision is made according to the surgical technique used. If the eye is phakic, a routine phaco or extracapsular cataract extraction (ECCE) procedure is performed and the IOL (power calculated according to biometry) planned for the patient is inserted into the capsular bag (▶ Fig. 23.1). The incision is then enlarged to 5 to 5.50 mm. The anterior chamber is filled with viscoelastic and the implant is also coated with viscoelastic (▶ Fig. 23.2). It is then grasped by the loops or the base of the loop, taking care not to touch the lens optic itself (▶ Fig. 23.3). It is inserted into the sulcus as a piggyback IOL with the posterior mirror (ring shaped) pointing toward the surgeon (▶ Fig. 23.4, ▶ Fig. 23.5). It is confirmed that the pupil on the operated eye is central. In case of an eccentric pupil, a pupilloplasty may be needed. A peripheral iridectomy is then done surgically (yttrium aluminum garnet laser should not be used). All the viscoelastic is removed and the incision is sutured.

Postoperative care is similar to that of a regular cataract extraction except that a closer watch is kept for anterior synechiae and IOP spike. Post-op tests are carried out at days 1, 2, 7, and 30, and 3, 6, and 12 months. The centration and position of the lens are checked for and the patient is refracted for distance and near uncorrected and best corrected visual acuity using the ETDRS chart (each eye separately). Postoperative specular microscopy is done.

23.5 Results

The initial outcomes are encouraging and a trial with larger number of patients recruited and a longer follow-up is being planned. Proper patient recruitment is a key factor in ensuring good outcomes as in every other case. The inclusion criteria for our pilot trial of the LMI-SI (OriLens) included patients with bilateral AMD (dry type, wet type, scar stage) or other similar macular lesions where the visual acuity ranged between 20/60 and 20/600 in each eye and improved for distance and/or near when tested with a × 2.5 magnification using an external telescope. Presence of any other systemic or ocular diseases (other than cataract/pseudophakia, AMD, or another macular lesion) excluded them, as also any other previous eye surgery other than cataract. Only those patients who were easy to communicate with, responsible, and understood his or her condition, who knew the risks and potential benefits involved, and who were highly motivated to read and improve visual capabilities were included. It was made sure that they understood that they would have to be available for follow-up of 1 year post-op. All the patients signed an informed consent. All other patients were excluded, as also those patients in whom the fellow eye suffers from medical problems, which would not

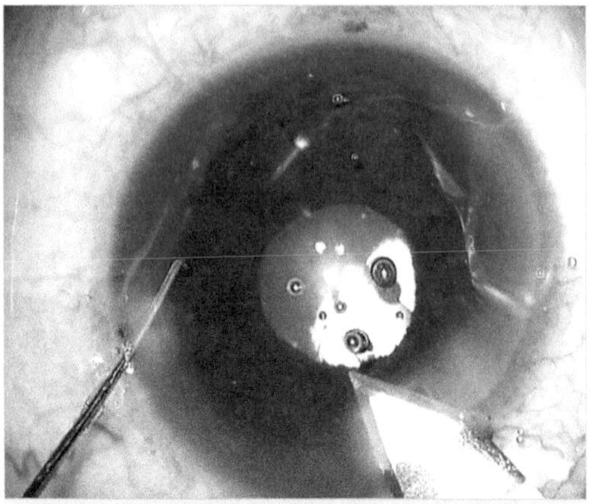

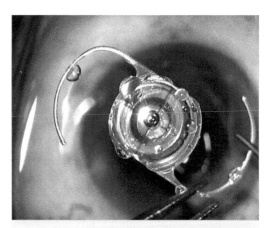

Fig. 23.1 A conventional foldable intraocular lens in the bag after performing cataract surgery.

Fig. 23.2 The LMI-SI (OriLens) is seen.

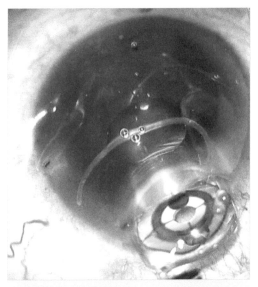

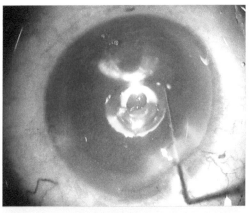

Fig. 23.4 On-table photograph showing the LMI-SI (OriLens) well centered with a clear cornea.

Fig. 23.3 The LMI-SI (OriLens) has been coated with viscoelastic and inserted through the clear corneal incision that has been extended just enough to allow implantation.

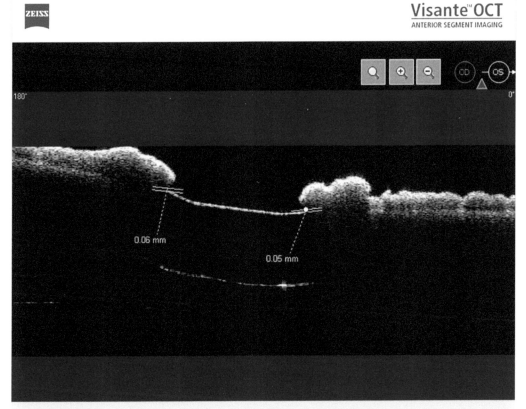

Fig. 23.5 The anterior segment optical coherence tomography showing the LMI-SI (OriLens) in the sulcus above the in-the-bag implanted intraocular lens.

enable the patient to use his peripheral vision, for example, those with glaucoma or retinitis pigmentosa.

23.6 Advantages of the LMI-SI

The advantages that the LMI-SI (OriLens) offers as compared to other available intraocular telescopic devices are many. It can be implanted in both eyes and it is surgeon friendly. It is a simple and safe surgery and can be performed by any cataract surgeon. It does not lie close to the corneal endothelium and hence chances of damage to the corneal endothelium are very low. It also offers a quick recovery for the patients who do not need prolonged and complicated postoperative training sessions for visual rehabilitation. It preserves part of the peripheral vision while magnifying the central field. It is also complementary to all other retinal treatments (injections, lasers, etc.) and can also be used for other retinal diseases.

Another big advantage of this IOL is the fact that it is placed in the sulcus over another IOL. As we know, a large majority of AMD patients may have already undergone cataract surgery with IOL implantation before presenting to the treating doctor. In such a case, it is still possible to offer the patient the opportunity of visual rehabilitation without having to undergo a complicated procedure such as explantation of the existing IOL and reimplantation of another telescopic device. As the LMI-SI (OriLens) can be easily placed in the sulcus, surgery is simple and it is also a one-lens-fit-all situation as the previously placed IOL in the bag takes care of the refractive error of the patient. Hence, the same LMI-SI (OriLens) can be offered to all patients irrespective of the biometric calculation of IOL power.

23.7 Key Pearls

- The telescopic IOLs are especially useful in cases with central vision loss as in cases with macular degeneration.
- The telescopic IOL is placed in the sulcus above the normal capsular bag–IOL implantation.
- The telescopic IOL acts by magnifying the central image on the retina, whereas the peripheral vision is unaltered. It thus facilitates the patients with central vision loss to apprehend images.

23.8 Financial Disclosures

Isaac Lipshitz has a financial interest in the LMI-SI (OriLens). None of the other authors have any financial interests relevant to the products or procedures mentioned here.

Videos

Video 23.1 Superman returns. The video demonstrates the mechanism of action of telescopic intraocular lens and its method of implantation with various benefits for patients with AMD.

References

[1] Hengerer FH, Artal P, Kohnen T, Conrad-Hengerer I. Initial clinical results of a new telescopic IOL implanted in patients with dry age-related macular degeneration. J Refract Surg. 2015; 31(3):158–162
[2] Agarwal A, Lipshitz I, Jacob S, et al. Mirror telescopic intraocular lens for age-related macular degeneration: design and preliminary clinical results of the Lipshitz macular implant. J Cataract Refract Surg. 2008; 34(1):87–94

Index

Note: Page numbers set **bold** or *italic* indicate headings or figures, respectively.

Index